PHARMACOLOGY - RESEARCH, SAFETY TESTING AND REGULATION

VANCOMYCIN

BIOSYNTHESIS, CLINICAL USES AND ADVERSE EFFECTS

PHARMACOLOGY - RESEARCH, SAFETY TESTING AND REGULATION

Additional books in this series can be found on Nova's website
under the Series tab.

Additional E-books in this series can be found on Nova's website
under the E-book tab.

PHARMACOLOGY - RESEARCH, SAFETY TESTING AND REGULATION

VANCOMYCIN

BIOSYNTHESIS, CLINICAL USES AND ADVERSE EFFECTS

ABU GAFAR HOSSION
EDITOR

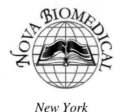

New York

Library of Congress Cataloging-in-Publication Data

ISBN: 978-1-62948-559-1

Published by Nova Science Publishers, Inc. † New York

Contents

Preface

News reports in bristle with the tales of many community acquired
bacterial infections that lead to serious hospitalization. The drug of last resort
for these infections is vancomycin; a FDA approved glycopeptide antibiotic
for the treatment several bacterial infections, including infections caused by
susceptible *Staphylococcus, Streptococcus,* Enterococcus, and diphtheroid
organisms. Around the world in 1997, initial reports of reduced vancomycin
susceptibility in clinical isolates of *Staphylococcus aureus* generated
significant concern in the medical community. There has been uncertainty
regarding optimal laboratory test and the clinical relevance of reduced
vancomycin susceptibility in *S. aureus*, changes in Clinical and Laboratory
Standards Institute (CLSI) breakpoints for vancomycin against *S. aureus*, and
increasing concern regarding the efficacy of vancomycin for the treatment of
infection due to *Gram-positive* bacteria such as *S. aureous*. Vancomycin can
be administered either intravenously or orally but to treat systemic infections
vancomycin must be administered intravenously. Identifying the changes in
genome content or espression which are associated with the acquisition of the
different types of vancomycin resistance is an important step in the process of
understanding the molecular basis of resistance, and has the potential to
provide leads both for new drug targets and for diagnostic biomarkers.
However, as vancomycin has a slow bactericidal activity, clinicians have to
adequately prescribe vancomycin, to avoid acquisition of resistance under
therapy and facilitate the cure.

Chapter 1 - For many years vancomycin has been an effect part of our
antibiotic armamentarium, remaining the first-line therapy for patients infected
with methicillin-resistant *Staphylococcus aureus*. However, settling on a dose

that optimizes efficacy and minimizes toxicity has also plagued this agent since becoming commercially available. In 2009, consensus recommendations were published acknowledging the pharmacodynamic parameter most associated with efficacy was the area-under-the-curve/minimum inhibitory concentration (AUC/MIC) ratio, but, instead of calculating the AUC, recommended vancomycin trough monitoring as a useful surrogate. Evidence published since 2009 has suggested the higher trough goals recommended in the consensus review may be leading to higher rates of vancomycin-associated nephrotoxicity, and no benefit in clinical outcomes has been found. Meanwhile, post-consensus data surrounding the AUC/MIC has continued to be promising in terms of safety and clinical outcomes. This chapter sets out to examine some of the clinical evidence surrounding current vancomycin trough goals and achieving goal AUC/MIC ratios; could the authors achieve clinical success with lower troughs?

Chapter 2 - Vancomycin resistance in Gram-positive bacteria can be classified as intermediate or high-level according to the differing susceptibilities that strains exhibit towards the antibiotic. Identifying the changes in genome content or expression which are associated with the acquisition of the different types of vancomycin resistance is an important step in the process of understanding the molecular basis of resistance, and has the potential to provide leads both for new drug targets and for diagnostic biomarkers. In this chapter the authors review the use of comparative and functional genomics approaches for addressing the questions: which adaptations in gene expression are important for determining the level of vancomycin susceptibility, and how do these produce the resultant phenotype? The picture that emerges is one where the acquisition of a small number of specific enzyme activities markedly reduces susceptibility, while a complex network of more generalised cellular mechanisms can be combined to produce low or intermediate effects.

Chapter 3 - Vancomycin is frequently used for the treatment of serious gram-positive infections involving methicillin-resistant *Staphylococcus aureus* (MRSA). It is also used for the treatment of infections caused by gram-positive microorganisms in patients with serious allergies to beta-lactam antibiotics and for the treatment of pseudomembranous colitis caused by the bacterium *Clostridium difficile*. Although early use of vancomycin was associated with nephrotoxicity and ototoxicity, it appears that impurities in early formulations were responsible, at least in part, for these toxic effects. To treat systemic infections, vancomycin must be administered intravenously. The intramuscular route is not used due to possible tissue necrosis. Vancomycin is not absorbed when it is orally administered, and this administration route is only used for the treatment of pseudomembranous colitis. The serum vancomycin concentration-time profile is complex and has been described with one-, two-, and three-compartment pharmacokinetic models. In patients with normal renal function, the terminal half-life ranges from 6 to 12 hours and the volume of distribution ranges from 0.4 to 1 L/kg. Several studies have indicated that vancomycin is a time-dependent (concentration-independent) killer of gram-positive pathogens, and that the best determinant of efficacy is the ratio of the area under the serum drug concentration-versus-time curve and the minimum inhibitory concentration (AUC/MIC). An AUC/MIC ratio equal to or above 400 has been recommended as target to achieve clinical effectiveness. Different vancomycin initial dosing schedules have been recommended for adults with impaired renal function, pediatric patients and neonates. Subsequent dosing should be adjusted based on serum vancomycin levels, using the AUC/MIC ratio as target, or trough concentrations as a surrogate marker for AUC when multiple serum vancomycin concentrations are not available to determine the AUC. In this sense, current recommendations have increased the so-called therapeutic range for trough levels from 5-10 mg/L to 10-15 mg/L and 15-20 mg/L, depending on the nature of the infection to be treated.

Chapter 4 - Antibiotics are routinely used for the decontamination of cardiovascular homografts. This step of bioburden reduction is critical, because manipulation during tissue recovery and processing, as well as environmental factors, may introduce contaminants to the homografts. As the consequences of implanting culture-positive homografts are potentially life-threatening, stringent measures are taken to eliminate microbial transmission to recipients. This includes the application of aseptic techniques in tissue processing, and antibiotic decontamination of homografts prior to long-term storage in liquid nitrogen vapour.

Usually, to target a diverse spectrum of endemic micro-organisms isolated from tissues, a cocktail of different antibiotics are utilised. In 2011, a collation of heart valve processing practices from 24 international heart valve banks in North America, Europe, Australasia and South Africa revealed that vancomycin is one of the most commonly used antibiotics in cardiovascular homograft banking. 62.5% of the banks included vancomycin of concentration 50-500 ug/ml in their antibiotic cocktail. Antibiotic regimens were validated by individual banks prior to implementation, to ensure that the antibiotic combination, incubation temperature and condition, yielded optimal bactericidal effect. The test systems used to detect microbial contamination of the homografts were also validated to ensure the results were not compromised by the presence of residual antibiotics. At the author's tissue bank, vancomycin is preferred, due to its broad spectrum and stability. This article briefly presents findings on the international banks' bioburden reduction practices and discusses the emerging importance of vancomycin in cardiovascular homograft banking.

Chapter 5 - Common and uncommon vancomycin adverse effects have been demonstrated here. Vancomycin is thought to be associated with a high rate of adverse events, mainly because most of tolerance studies were conduct with early preparation containing impurities. Vancomycin is known to be venotoxic, and is frequently associated with thrombosis, especially if vancomycin is administered through a peripheral catheter. When administered through central venous catheter, thrombosis are uncommon, but could be observed in association with superior cava syndrome. Reported in up to 11% of patients, infusion-related reactions due to histamine release (red-man or red-neck syndrome) represents the most frequent side effect of vancomycin, which occurs when the duration of vancomycin perfusion is less than one hour. In recent studies, vancomycin-associated nephrotoxicity occurs in approximately 5% of patients, and is associated to high plasmatic levels (> 15 mg/L), concomitant use of nephrotoxic agents, long treatment durations, and possibly intermittent infusions. If the role of vancomycin in ototoxicity is still debated, a reversible hearing loss may occur in 12% of patients, mainly in the elderly. Other vancomycin-induced adverse events include allergic reactions (2-3%), neutropenia (1-2%) and thrombocytopenia. In addition of targeting efficient plasmatic rates, measurement of trough plasmatic concentration may reduce the incidence of vancomycin-related side effects.

Chapter 6 - The clinical use of vancomycin in methicillin-resistant *S. aureus* or coagulase-negative staphylococci bacteremia, catheter-related bacteremia and endocarditis has been developed in this chapter. These methicillin-resistant *S. aureus* or coagulase-negative staphylococci bacteremia, catheter-related bacteremia and endocarditis pathogens are mainly related with health-care associated infections, and particularly catheter-related infections. Coagulase-negative staphylococci are considered to be less virulent than *S. aureus*, as they are less frequently associated with complications and mortality. Methicillin-resistant staphylococci isolated from blood cultures are usually susceptible to vancomycin with a minimal inhibitory concentration (MIC) ≤ 2 µg/mL for *S. aureus* and ≤ 4µg/mL for coagulase-negative staphylococci. Vancomycin remained the treatment of choice of such infections. However, as vancomycin has a slow bactericidal activity, clinicians have to adequately prescribe vancomycin, to avoid acquisition of resistance under therapy and facilitate the cure. Several reports indicate that in the range of susceptibility, high MICs (i.e between 1.5 and 2 µg/mL for *S. aureus*) are associated with a higher risk of relapse or death. Area under the curve (AUC)/MIC is the stronger predictive pharmacokinetic parameter for vancomycin efficacy in patients with bacteremia. An AUC/MIC ratio ≥400 is considered to be adequate to obtain clinical effectiveness, whereas trough serum concentration at the equilibrium is the most accurate method to evaluate the vancomycin effectiveness. A trough serum of 20 mg/L allows obtaining an AUC/MIC ratio ≥400, even if the MIC of the isolate is close to the susceptibility breakpoint. Vancomycin has to be administered intravenously, through a central venous catheter (a peripheral access could be used during the first days of therapy), with a dosage of 15 mg/kg/d twice a day. Uncomplicated methicillin-resistant *S. aureus* or coagulase-negative staphylococci bacteremia requires at least 14 days of vancomycin therapy. The duration of the therapy should be prolonged in uncomplicated *S. aureus* bacteremia if patients have diabetes, or receive immunosuppressive drugs. In patients with *S. aureus* catheter-related bacteremia, the catheter has always to be removed, whereas vancomycin lock therapy can be used in patients with uncomplicated methicillin-resistant coagulase-negative staphylococci catheter-related infections, in conjunction with systemic vancomycin therapy. For vancomycin lock therapy, vancomycin is combined with heparin and instilled into each catheter lumen, each day during 14 days. In patients with complicated catheter-related bacteremia and native valve endocarditis, the duration of the vancomycin therapy has to be prolonged to 6 weeks, and has to be combined with gentamicin during 3-5 days. In patients with prosthetic valve endocarditis, vancomycin has to be combined with gentamicin during 14 days, and with rifampin during the 6 weeks.

Chapter 7 - The authors have developed in this chapter the clinical use of vancomycin in MRSA hospital-acquired pneumonia. MRSA hospital-acquired pneumonia is associated with a significant morbidity and long hospital stays, particularly in intensive care units for patients with ventilator-associated pneumonia (VAP). Patients with VAP should have vancomycin as empirical therapy, immediately after the bronchoalveolar lavage, if MRSA is suspected (patient known to be MRSA carrier, late VAP). Vancomycin has to be administered intravenously through a central venous catheter with a dosage of 15 mg/kg/d twice a day. The dose has to be reduced for patients with renal failure. Monitoring serum concentration is required to optimize vancomycin therapy. Linezolid may be more effective than vancomycin, as suggested by two randomized controlled double-blind trials, as a possible consequence of vancomycin poor penetration into the lung. Linezolid could also be used to terminate the therapy in patients treated with vancomycin for MRSA VAP, if the central venous catheter is lost. Two weeks of therapy are usually sufficient to treat MRSA VAP.

Chapter 8 - In this chapter the clinical use of vancomycin in methicillin-resistant *S. aureus* or coagulase-negative staphylococci bone and joint infection (BJI) has been developed. BJI is one of the most difficult-to-treat infectious diseases, especially if an implant, such as osteosynthesis or joint prosthesis, is localized at the site of infection. These pathogens are the most frequent causative agents of BJI, particularly in postoperative or posttraumatic BJI. Staphylococci have the ability to modify their phenotype, by producing biofilm or small colony variants, which are particularly associated with chronic infection and relapse. In postoperative or in posttraumatic BJI, vancomycin has not to be used before optimal surgery (lavage and debridement, with implant retention or explantation), that: (i) allows the microbiological diagnosis; (ii) reduces the bacterial inoculum; (iii) eradicates sequestra in which staphylococci are embedded in biofilm; and (iv) facilitates bone vascularization and the diffusion of antimicrobials. Vancomycin has to be administered intravenously, through a central venous catheter (a peripheral access could be used during the first days of therapy), with a dosage of 15 mg/kg/d twice a day. As vancomycin activity is considered to be time-dependent, some data support the use of continuous infusion of vancomycin, to achieve a time under MIC (*t*/MIC) close to 100%. Targeting methicillin-resistant *S. aureus* or coagulase-negative staphylococci, vancomycin has to be combined with another active drug, and especially an oral drug, which has a high biodisponibility and bone penetration such as fluoroquinolones, clindamycin or rifampin. Rifampin has to be preferred in patients with implant-associated BJI. If possible, vancomycin could be switched after 2 weeks of therapy, to use a combination of two oral active drugs. If not, the regiment including vancomycin has to be prolonged until 6-24 weeks, depending on the clinical presentation. In these patients, it is crucial to monitor vancomycin trough serum concentration and to be aware of putative vancomycin toxicity.

In: Vancomycin   ISBN: 978-1-62948-559-1
Editor: Abu Gafar Hossion   © 2013 Nova Science Publishers, Inc.

Chapter 1

Pharmacodynamic Dosing of Vancomycin: Concepts and Clinical Evidence

Ryan P. Moenster, Pharm.D., BCPS (AQ ID)[*1]
and Travis W. Linneman, Pharm.D., BCPS[2]

[1]Associate Professor of Pharmacy Practice
St. Louis College of Pharmacy
Clinical Pharmacy Specialist – Infectious Diseases
VA St. Louis Health Care System – John Cochran Division, UK
[2]Assistant Professor of Pharmacy Practice
St. Louis College of Pharmacy
Clinical Pharmacy Specialist – Internal Medicine
VA St. Louis Health Care System – John Cochran Division, UK

Abstract

For many years vancomycin has been an effective part of our antibiotic armamentarium, remaining the first-line therapy for patients infected with methicillin-resistant *Staphylococcus aureus*. However, settling on a dose that optimizes efficacy and minimizes toxicity has also plagued this agent since becoming commercially available. In 2009,

* Corresponding Authors e-mail: Ryan.Moenster@stlcop.edu and Travis.Linneman@stlcop.edu.

consensus recommendations were published acknowledging the pharmacodynamic parameter most associated with efficacy was the area-under-the-curve/minimum inhibitory concentration (AUC/MIC) ratio, but, instead of calculating the AUC, recommended vancomycin trough monitoring as a useful surrogate. Evidence published since 2009 has suggested the higher trough goals recommended in the consensus review may be leading to higher rates of vancomycin-associated nephrotoxicity, and no benefit in clinical outcomes has been found. Meanwhile, post-consensus data surrounding the AUC/MIC has continued to be promising in terms of safety and clinical outcomes. This chapter sets out to examine some of the clinical evidence surrounding current vancomycin trough goals and achieving goal AUC/MIC ratios; could we achieve clinical success with lower troughs?

Keywords: Vancomycin, Antibiotics, Pharmacokinetics

A Brief History of Vancomycin

Since its discovery in the 1950s, vancomycin has played a part in saving countless lives worldwide, but has also remained a source of confusion and controversy. Vancomycin was first identified in soil samples obtained from Borneo in 1952. Scientists at Eli Lily identified a compound, originally named "compound 05865", produced by *Streptomyces orientalis* isolated from soil samples. After determining that the compound was active against many gram-positive organisms, including penicillin-resistant strains of *Staphylococcus aureus*, it became evident that clinical trials were warranted; vancomycin ultimately became commercially available in 1958 [1,2].

Originally tagged with the nickname "Mississippi Mud" (due to its brown color), early vancomycin preparations were thought to be impure; these visual impurities were believed to be the cause of adverse effects (notably venous irritation, chills, rash, and ototoxicity). This perception of toxicity associated with these early preparations, and the subsequent release of methicillin and cephalothin also in 1958, led to vancomycin being reserved for patients with severe β-lactam allergies, or those infected with bacteria resistant to newer antibiotics [1].

The 1980s saw the advent of wide-spread, clinically relevant infections with methicillin-resistant *S. aureus* (MRSA), and a subsequent exponential increase in the use of vancomycin. Vancomycin has remained highly effective against MRSA; however, with increased rates of MRSA infection, and the subsequent increase in vancomycin usage, less susceptible strains of *S. aureus* have emerged. The first reported cases of reduced susceptibility to vancomycin in *S. aureus* isolates came from Japan in 1997, with resistance among enterococcal isolates appearing earlier in 1986 [1]. With the emergence of resistance and intermediate susceptibility, more attention was paid to the pharmacokinetics and pharmacodynamics of vancomycin; was the current dosing adequate?

Vancomycin Pharmacokinetics and Pharmacodynamics

The initial dosing of vancomycin was developed based on early *in vitro* and human pharmacokinetic studies. Initially, vancomycin was found to be bactericidal against *Streptococcus pyogenes* and *Micrococcus pyogenes* var. *aureus* (now classified as *Staphylococcus aureus*) at concentrations of 0.67 and 2 mcg/mL respectively. [3] Corresponding pharmacokinetic studies conducted at the time evaluated serum and urine vancomycin levels after 100 mg was administered intravenously (IV) every six to eight hours in healthy patients; serum concentrations six hours after a dose of 100 mg was administered ranged from 0.5-1 mcg/mL. While these levels seem woefully inadequate by today's standards, these authors also report 3 cases of patients cured by 100 mg of vancomycin given every eight hours, and one cured with 50 mg every 6 hours [4].

A later study, published in the *Mayo Clinic Proceedings* in 1956, evaluated serum vancomycin levels of healthy volunteers given a single dose of 500 mg IV. In the eight volunteers, serum vancomycin concentrations 24-hours after a single dose of 500 mg averaged 0.7 mcg/mL. Five subjects with active infection were also included in a subset of this analysis; serum vancomycin concentrations were measured after the antibiotic had been administered every six to eight hours for 2-3 days. Serum concentrations ranged from 6.4 – 10.5 mcg/mL in patients after the ninth dose of vancomycin was administered [5]. Based on what was known regarding minimum inhibitory concentrations (MIC) for streptococci and staphylococci, it appeared these trough concentrations were more than adequate for bactericidal activity, and troughs in the range of 5 – 10 mcg/mL were considered therapeutic [2,5].

The first studies evaluating the pharmacodynamics (PD) of vancomycin in a murine model were presented in 1987. This evaluation demonstrated that the area-under-the-curve (AUC) was a more important parameter at determining efficacy against methicillin-susceptible *S. aureus* (MSSA) and MRSA than time above the MIC, the PD parameter most associated with efficacy for β-lactams [6, 7]. A later study of neutropenic mice with induced thigh infections further determined that the ratio of 24-hour AUC to organism MIC (AUC/MIC) ratio was the pharmacokinetic-pharmacodynamic (PK-PD) parameter that best correlated with vancomycin efficacy [6].

Since this time, the AUC/MIC ratio has been studied in an effort to better determine what specific AUC/MIC value was most-associated with vancomycin efficacy. One of the seminal works in this area was published by Moise-Broder et al., in 2004, in which 108 patients with documented *S. aureus* nosocomial pneumonia and treated with >72 hours of vancomycin had AUC/MIC ratios calculated to determine which level was most associated with clinical and microbiologic efficacy. Patients with vancomycin AUC/MIC ratios >350 were 7-times more likely to achieve clinical success (OR 7.19, 95% CI 1.91-27.3; $p<0.05$), and those with AUC/MIC ratios >400 had a median time to organism eradication of 10 days; patients with an AUC/MIC <400 demonstrated a median time to respiratory culture clearance in excess of 30 days (only 20% of patients in this group actually demonstrated organism clearance) [8].

It became apparent after the work by Moise-Broder et al., that previously accepted vancomycin trough goals of 5 – 10 mcg/mL would likely not achieve AUC/MIC ratios >350-400 [9] In 2005, the American Thoracic Society and Infectious Diseases Society of America published guidelines for the management of adults with hospital-acquired, ventilator-associated, and healthcare-associated pneumonia. Citing previous work demonstrating vancomycin penetration into the lungs that was, on average, 41% of serum levels after 12 hours, and taking into consideration optimal AUC/MIC ratios were likely >350-400, the guidelines advocated a goal trough range of 15-20 mcg/mL; however, this new trough range was based largely on clinical opinion [8,10, 11].

Vancomycin: A Consensus Review

In an effort to better identify what should be targeted as a therapeutic goal during vancomycin treatment and how serum concentrations should be monitored, the Infectious Diseases Society of America, the American Society of Health-System Pharmacists, and the Society of Infectious Disease Pharmacists published consensus recommendations in 2009. This review discusses pharmacokinetic and pharmacodynamic properties of vancomycin, pharmacokinetic and pharmacodynamic monitoring parameters associated with vancomycin use, the impact of dosing strategies on pharmacokinetic and pharmacodynamic parameters of vancomycin, and therapeutic drug monitoring of vancomycin, including optimal trough values. The review also covers potential vancomycin toxicity and the role of therapeutic vancomycin drug monitoring on mitigating these toxicities. Key recommendations and conclusions from this consensus review related to goal pharmacokinetic/pharmacodynamic parameters of vancomycin can be found in table 1 [9].

Table 1. Key Recommendations and Conclusions from the Vancomycin Consensus Review: Goal Pharmacokinetic/Pharmacodynamic Parameters [9]

- Vancomycin does not display concentration dependent bacterial killing.
- An AUC/MIC ratio of ≥ 400 has been advocated to achieve clinical effectiveness with vancomycin. The AUC/MIC ratio is a predictive pharmacokinetic parameter for vancomycin.
- Because it may be difficult to obtain multiple serum vancomycin concentrations to determine the AUC for a patient, trough serum vancomycin values are the most accurate and practical method for monitoring vancomycin effectiveness.
- Vancomycin trough levels of > 10 mg/L are recommended to avoid the development of resistance.
- Vancomycin trough levels of 15-20 mg/L are recommended because of the potential to improve penetration, increase the probability of optimal target serum vancomycin concentrations, and improve clinical outcomes for complicated infections (bacteremia, endocarditis, osteomyelitis, meningitis, and hospital-acquired pneumonia).
- Trough serum vancomycin levels of 15-20 mg/L should achieve an AUC/MIC of ≥ 400 in most patients if the MIC is ≤ 1 mg/L.
- Alternative therapies for infections caused by bacteria with a vancomycin MIC ≥ 2 mg/L should be considered as conventional dosing is unlikely to result in an AUC/MIC of ≥ 400 in patients with normal renal function.
- Continuous infusion regimens are unlikely to substantially improve patient outcome (compared to intermittent dosing).

The authors conclude that the PK-PD parameter most-associated with beneficial therapeutic outcome is an AUC/MIC ratio ≥400, but, given the difficulty in measuring vancomycin AUC, the review recommends vancomycin troughs as a more practical surrogate for the AUC. Based on these recommendations and data presented in the review, many clinicians target vancomycin trough values of 15-20 mg/L, especially for patients that are seriously ill or have difficult to treat infections. While these recommendations note that most patients will require 15-20 mg/kg based on ABW given every 8 – 12 hours to achieve goal trough levels (and subsequently AUC/MIC ratio goals), it is important to note that the review also recommends individual pharmacokinetic adjustments and verification of trough levels. The review further notes that most available nomograms, at the time of consensus development, were not developed to target vancomycin levels of 15-20 mg/L. And while the weight based dosing is noted above, it is also important to note that these recommendations suggest doses of 15-20mg/kg given every 8 – 12 hours will be required, but do not provide specific recommendations on calculating a dose, or how to choose an appropriate dosing interval for a patient. Additionally, while pharmacokinetic adjustments are recommended, specific methods or strategies of adjustment are not reviewed or recommended. Key recommendations and conclusions from this consensus review related to vancomycin dosing to achieve recommended pharmacokinetic/pharmacodynamics parameters can be found in table 2 [9].

Table 2. Key Recommendations and Conclusions from the Vancomycin Consensus Review: Achieving Pharmacokinetic/Pharmacodynamic Parameters [9]

- Actual body weight should be utilized to calculate initial vancomycin doses.
- A loading dose of 25-30 mg/kg of ABW can be considered for rapid attainment of target trough concentrations in seriously ill patients.
- Vancomycin doses of 15-20 mg/kg given every 8 – 12 hours are required for patients with normal renal function to achieve suggested trough levels with an MIC ≤ 1 mg/L.
- Individual pharmacokinetic adjustments and verification of serum trough levels are recommended.

This review also highlights the inconsistency in available data regarding the relationship of vancomycin levels (both peaks and troughs) and potential toxicity. Based on available data, however, monitoring of trough levels in an effort to prevent prolonged troughs of > 20 mg/L is pertinent. The safety of maintaining trough levels between 15 – 20 mg/L is not well supported with data, and some data suggest that these troughs may contribute to increased rates of vancomycin related nephrotoxicity. Frequent (at least once or twice weekly) monitoring of signs or symptoms of vancomycin nephrotoxicity is therefore recommended [9].

Clinical Benefit from Higher Trough Goals

Limited data has been published evaluating clinical outcomes with the higher vancomycin goal troughs endorsed by the consensus review. These recommendations are primarily based on evidence supporting an AUC/MIC of ≥ 400, coupled with PK-PD evaluations/simulations demonstrating likelihood of achieving this goal with varying vancomycin regimens and serum trough values; even at the time the consensus review was developed there was almost no published evidence correlating better clinical outcomes and higher vancomycin troughs [9].

Jeffres et al., evaluated predictors, specifically vancomycin pharmacokinetic indexes including the use of higher vancomycin troughs (15-20 mg/L), in a retrospective cohort of patients with healthcare associated MRSA pneumonia confirmed by bronchoalveolar lavage. One-hundred two patients were included in the investigation with an overall mortality rate of 31.4% (32 patients). Non-survivors were more likely to have end-stage renal disease requiring hemodialysis, to have higher acute physiology and chronic health evaluation (APACHE) II scores, and to require mechanical ventilation and vasopressor support as compared to survivors; no relationship between vancomycin troughs and estimated AUC values and survivors or non-survivors was found. Further, a secondary analysis comparing patient groups with vancomycin steady-state concentrations < 15 mcg/mL compared to those with concentrations ≥ 15 mcg/mL was completed. Despite a mean trough concentrations of 9.4 ± 3.2 mcg/mL and 20.4 ± 3.2 mcg/mL between these groups, and a mean AUC values of 318 ± 111 and 418 ± 158, the hospital mortality rate was not statistically different (29.4% and 35.3% respectively).[12]

While this study did not corroborate previous investigations linking higher AUC values to vancomycin treatment success, it is important to note some limitations. Minimum inhibitory concentrations of the identified MRSA isolates were not available resulting in an evaluation of AUC values only and not AUC/MIC values and clinical success. Further, while mean vancomycin trough concentrations between groups were well separated, stratification by vancomycin trough concentration included 27 patients with vancomycin troughs < 10 mc/mL, 35 with trough concentrations of 10 − 15 mcg/mL, 17 with trough concentrations of 15.1 − 20 mcg/mL and 16 with concentrations > 20 mcg/mL. Additionally, mean AUC values had large standard deviations and subsequently overlapping values/standard deviation ranges. Finally, lacking a power calculation, the results are potentially subject to a Type II error.

Kullar et al., characterized risk factors for vancomycin failure in the setting of MRSA bacteremia, including PK-PD factors of vancomycin use. Patients with documented MRSA bacteremia and vancomycin therapy for at least 72 hours were evaluated as a retrospective cohort. Utilizing initial vancomycin steady-state trough levels and estimated AUC values were the PK-PD factors included as potential predictors in the logistic regression model.

Three hundred twenty patients were included, of whom more than half met the authors' definition of vancomycin failure. Logistic regression identified infective endocarditis, nosocomial-acquired infection, initial vancomycin trough < 15 mg/L, and vancomycin MIC > 1 mg/L as independent predictors of failure of therapy. An initial vancomycin trough of < 15 mg/L had an AOR of 2.00 (95% CI, 1.25-3.22) and an isolate with a vancomycin MIC > 1 mg/L had an AOR of 1.52 (95% CI, 1.09 − 2.49). Analysis of AUC data utilizing a Classification and Regression Tree analysis (CART) demonstrated that patients with AUC/MIC ratios of < 421 had significantly higher failure rates than those with an AUC/MIC ratio of > 421 (61.2% vs 48.6%).[13]

Similar to previous data, this data is not without limitations. However, by identifying initial vancomycin trough of < 15 mg/L as an independent risk factor for vancomycin therapy failure, this evaluation generally supports the consensus review recommendation of targeting troughs of at least 15 mg/L (15-20 mg/L) for complicated or serious infections. Additionally, the findings of significantly higher failure rates of vancomycin in patients not achieving an AUC/MIC ratio of > 421 is generally consistent with previous findings (except that of Jeffers et al., described above) and supports the recommendation of targeting an AUC/MIC ratio of at least 400.

Higher Trough Goals: More Harm than Good?

There has also been building concern that targeting higher vancomycin trough levels may result in an increased incidence of vancomycin-associated nephrotoxicity. The review noted that data available at the time of review development was limited, with published data being conflicting. Additionally, the review highlighted that this issue has been complicated by the history of impurities present in early vancomycin formulations potentially contributing to adverse events, including nephrotoxicity, varying definitions of nephrotoxicity utilized in investigations of this issue, patients treated with vancomycin often requiring concurrent treatment with other nephrotoxic agents, and difficulty in determining specific timing of events and cause-and-effect relationships. These confounders, along with the fact that patients requiring vancomycin therapy may seriously ill or medically unstable, have made evaluating the potential for vancomycin to be associated with nephrotoxicity, especially at higher trough levels, difficult [9].

An evaluation of vancomycin trough concentrations and the relationship between increased efficacy or toxicity in burn patients completed by Ackerman et al., found that renal toxicity may be correlated with duration of treatment, but not specifically to trough concentration. One limitation of this study in the context of considering the potential nephrotoxicity of vancomycin with trough levels of 15 – 20 mg/L is that the highest strata group of patients evaluated included all patients with trough values > 10 mg/L and was not specific to those with values > 15 mg/L [14].

In the previously described retrospective cohort evaluation by Kullar et al., the authors did not detect a significant difference in nephrotoxicity in vancomycin treated patients with steady-state concentrations of 15-20 mg/L when compared to groups with values < 10 or 10 – 14.9 mg/L. This study did, however, note a significantly different higher incidence of nephrotoxicity in those with trough values of > 20 mg/L as compared with the 15 – 20 mg/L group [13].

A separate evaluation published by Kullar et al., in 2012 evaluated the effects of targeting higher vancomycin trough levels on clinical outcomes, including rates of nephrotoxicity, comparing a matched cohort of patients with complicated MRSA bacteremia treated with vancomycin pre- and post-implementation of goal troughs of 15-20 mg/L. Among other results, this evaluation found that pre-implementation patients (targeting lower troughs) had a non-statistically significant lower rate of nephrotoxicity than those patients treated with higher trough goals (15% vs 18%, p=0.85) [15].

Horey, et al., examined the relationship of nephrotoxicity to vancomycin troughs in a veteran's population. In a retrospective analysis of 270 patients receiving vancomycin for 48 hours or more and having an evaluable vancomycin trough within 96 hours of initiation of therapy, maximum trough concentration had an OR of 1.14 (95% CI 1.09 − 1.20) of being associated with renal toxicity. Of note, documented hypotension and weight were also identified as significantly associated with renal toxicity with hypotension having the highest OR of 4.7 (95% CI 1.3 − 16.4). After stratifying vancomycin trough levels to ranges of 5-10 mg/L, 10.1 − 15 mg/L, 15.1 − 20 mg/L, 20.1 − 35 mg/L and > 35 mg/L, increasing trough values were associated with an elevated risk of developing nephrotoxicity. Rates of nephrotoxicity for the ranges above were 4.7%, 3.1%, 10.6% (15-20 mg/L), 23.6%, and 81.8% respectively [16].

An evaluation completed by Hall et al., examined the relationship of the consensus review weight-based dosing recommendations of at least 15mg/kg/dose and the development of renal toxicity. Patients receiving at least 48 hours of vancomycin were evaluated utilizing multivariable general linear mixed-effect model to identify predictors or associations for nephrotoxicity. This study found similar rates of nephrotoxicity development with vancomycin therapy among those treated with the consensus recommended dosing and those with lower dosing (24% vs 22%). Multivariate analysis further supported this conclusion with weight-based dosing of at least 15 mg/kg/dose not being identified as a predictor of renal toxicity. Those factors most associated with nephrotoxicity included vancomycin therapy for more than 15 days, trough vancomycin values > 20 mcg/ml, and age over 52 years [17].

A systematic review and meta-analysis published in 2013 by Hal, et al., attempted to further address the question of vancomycin trough value goals of 15 − 20 mg/L and the potential for vancomycin-induced nephrotoxicity. Initial searches identified 240 studies from 1996 − April 2012, of which 38 studies met review criteria and 15 were included for analysis. In a group of studies mostly including adults, after adjustments for covariates known to increase risk of nephrotoxicity, troughs of greater than or equal to 15 mg/L were associated with an OR for nephrotoxicity of 2.67 (95% CI 1.95 − 3.65) when compared to troughs maintained lower than 15 mg/L. Overall, this analysis concluded that the probability of nephrotoxicity while on vancomycin increased with the trough concentration and the duration of vancomycin therapy [18].

While data is conflicting, taken together, this information suggests a correlation of increasing risk of vancomycin related nephrotoxicity with increasing vancomycin troughs, especially at troughs > 20 mg/L. Additionally, the data generally states that the risk of renal toxicity related to vancomycin may increase with longer durations of therapy. These two relationships together may be especially important when considering patients that may require higher trough values for extended periods of time (i.e, those with endocarditis or osteomyelitis).

AUC/MIC Ratio or Trough Concentrations: Where Should the Focus Be?

The 2009 consensus review for the therapeutic monitoring of vancomycin has served to standardize goal vancomycin troughs for some serious infections and give clear recommendations as to the timing of appropriate troughs, but, as stated previously, many of these recommendations are based on expert opinion and not supported by large trials [9]. Also, as discussed previously, evidence supporting better clinical outcomes in patients in whom higher troughs are targeted is lacking, or, at best, conflicting. Several authors, however, have evaluated if attainment of goal AUC/MIC ratios improves mortality in patients with *S. aureus* bacteremia.

In 2012, Brown et al., retrospectively studied 50 patients treated with at least 48 hours of vancomycin for complicated bacteremia or infective endocarditis caused by MRSA. Patients with an AUC/MIC ratio <211 were found to have a >4-fold increase in attributable mortality; multivariate logistic regression identified only APACHE-II scores and AUC/MIC ratios <211 as independently associated with an increase in attributable mortality (AOR 1.24 [*P=0.04*] and 10.4 [*P=0.01*] respectively) [19]. The retrospective nature of this evaluation, and the fact that it was conducted at a single-center study before publication of the vancomycin guidelines, as well as the fact that calculated AUC/MIC break-point for a difference in mortality is well-below what the guidelines endorse targeting, are limitations as we assess the work.

More recently, Holmes et al., retrospectively studied 30-day all-cause mortality in 182 patients receiving vancomycin for *S.aureus* bacteremia. These authors first studied what difference, if any, attainment of an AUC/MIC ≥ 400 would have on mortality; a non-significant reduction of 8% in mortality was calculated. In addition to calculating the mortality difference at ≥ 400, a CART analysis was completed to determine an AUC/MIC break-point for all-cause mortality. An AUC/MIC break-point of 373 was calculated, and a statistically significant benefit in all-cause mortality was observed in patients who achieved an AUC/MIC ratio of $\geq$ 373 (71.6% vs. 84.3%; $P=0.043$). Additionally, multivariable logistic regression identified that patients achieving an AUC/MIC >373 had a significantly lower rate of 30-day all-cause mortality (OR 0.44, 95% CI 0.22-0.99; $P=0.049$). The authors also identified that the method of determining the organism MIC significantly impacted the AUC/MIC ratio; CART analysis revealing that, for patients with MICs determined by Etest, those with AUC/MIC ratios <211 had higher attributable mortality. As with the Brown et al., study, the retrospective nature does serve as a limitation, and achievement of the accepted AUC/MIC ratio goal of >400 was not associated with significant reduction in mortality [20].

Even though they are retrospective in nature, the previous two studies have demonstrated that a mortality benefit can be seen by achieving a particular AUC/MIC ratio, but, as shown in the previous section, a benefit has not been observed by targeting a particular vancomycin trough, and, in fact, higher trough goals may be associated with an increased risk of nephrotoxicity. Given this information, a relevant question becomes, by focusing on the AUC/MIC ratio rather than troughs, can we achieve similar rates of clinical cure, while reducing serum vancomycin concentrations and rates of nephrotoxicity? While little work has been done in this area to date, a recent study conducted by Le et al., did evaluate this questions in a simulated PK-PD model in pediatrics. Clinical data from 702 patients between the ages of 3 months and 18 years-old was used to develop a PK model; this validated PK model was then used in an 11,000 patient Monte Carlo simulation. At a simulated dose of 70 mg/kg/day, >85% of the patients achieved a goal AUC/MIC of >400, however, only 50% of patients would have achieved a trough concentration $\geq$ 15 mcg/mL [21]. Additionally, the authors determined age and SCr would play a major role in achieving the goal AUC/MIC ratio, observing that <75% of patients with a SCr <0.65 mg/dL would reach an AUC/MIC of >400. While theoretical in nature, this work does serve to demonstrate that troughs $\geq$ 15 mcg/mL may not be necessary to achieve an adequate AUC/MIC.

While the AUC is undoubtedly important, one cannot ignore the importance of the denominator, the MIC, in achieving an AUC/MIC ratio of $\geq$ 400. Patel et al., used Monte Carlo simulations to evaluate the probability of attaining goal AUC/MIC ratios for various doses of vancomycin, across different creatinine clearances (CrCls) and simulated MICs ranging from 0.5-2 mcg/mL. At the highest tested dose of vancomycin (4 gm/d), the probability of attaining the goal AUC/MIC ratio of >400 was only 57% if the *S. aureus* had an MIC of 2 mcg/mL; if 2gm/d was used to treat an isolate with an MIC of 2 mcg/mL, the probability of achieving the goal was 15% [22]. For example, if a patient was found to have an AUC of 500 and infected with a *S. aureus* isolate with an MIC of 0.5 mcg/mL, the AUC/MIC ratio would be 1000, over 2-times our goal of 400. However, if a patient had the same AUC, but was infected with an isolate with an MIC of 2 mcg/mL, the AUC/MIC ratio would 250, well below our goal. The data from Patel et al., serves as a helpful reminder that no matter what goal clinicians are trying to achieve, non-patient factors, such as the organism MIC, significantly impact the probability of achieving goal AUC/MIC ratios and positive clinical outcomes.

While the consensus review acknowledges the AUC/MIC ratio as the PK-PD parameter most associated with positive clinical outcomes in patients treated with vancomycin, the committee favored monitoring serum trough concentrations instead of calculating AUCs, however, retrospective data published after the consensus recommendations has shown that the higher trough goals are not associated with better clinical outcomes, and may cause higher rates of nephrotoxicity. Continuing the work of determining which parameters are most associated with positive clinical outcomes, authors such as Brown et al., and Holmes et al., have determined that AUC/MIC ratios can be correlated with mortality benefits, while Le et al., has shown in her model that the goal AUC/MIC ratio outlined in the consensus recommendations can be achieved with troughs below 15 mcg/mL. If one takes the recommendations from the consensus committee and factors-in the data that has been elucidated after the recommendations were published, it appears the most evidence-based approach to determining optimal vancomycin dosing would involve trough monitoring and the calculation of the AUC/MIC ratio.

Individualization of Doses: Calculating Doses, Estimating Troughs, and Estimating AUC

There are many validated models for completing vancomycin pharmacokinetic dosing model estimates, among them Matzke, Rodvold, Birt,

Burton, Ambrose and Bauer specific. These models are often utilized to develop vancomycin dosing regimens targeting specific vancomycin trough goals. The consensus recommendations cite difficulty in measuring AUC values as part of the justification for utilizing trough values. However, models also exist for estimating AUC values based on vancomycin kinetic parameters.

Given that the preferred vancomycin therapy target PK-PD parameter is AUC/MIC, it may be prudent to utilize both peak and trough estimate models, along with AUC estimate models, in order to develop and evaluate vancomycin regimens for specific patients. This is especially important in that, while vancomycin trough values correlate with AUC values, there is significant patient-to-patient variation in what AUC a specific vancomycin trough value may reflect or suggest. Consider the following example:

A 57 year old male being treated with vancomycin for a serious MRSA bacteremia. The MRSA vancomycin MIC is 1. The patient is 72 inches tall, 86 kg, with a serum creatinine of 0.83.

CrCl (Cockroft-Gault): 107 ml/min

$Vancomycin_{CL} = 80$ ml/min = 4.8 L/hr

Vd = 0.57 L/kg * 86kg = 49L

$Ke = 4.8$ L/h / 49 L = 0.098 h^{-1}

$t_{1/2} = 0.693/0.098 = 7$ hours

Consider a regimen of 1250mg q12h for this patient.

Utilizing the Sawchuk and Zaske model with an infusion time of 2 hours, the C_{max} results in an estimated peak of approximately 33.5 and a trough of 12.5 mg/L. However, estimating an AUC for the dosing interval results in a value of 230 for the each dosing interval, and a value of 460 for an entire day's dosing regimen. The regimen for this patient is then able to maintain an estimated target AUC of > 400 with a trough below 15 mg/L. Based on the data outlined above and recommendations of the consensus review, individualization of dose accounting for both estimated trough and AUC values may provide the opportunity to target appropriate pk/pd values with lower troughs.

Table 3. Selected Useful Pharmacokinetic Equations [23]

Estimated Vancomycin Clearance (mL/min/kg) = 0.695 x $\dfrac{(CrCl)}{(TBW)}$ + 0.05

Volume of Distribution (L): CrCl $\geq$ 60 mL/min: 0.57 L/kg x TBW
CrCl< 60 mL/min: 0.83 L/kg x TBW

Estimated Vancomycin Elimination Rate Constant (k_e): $\dfrac{Vancomycin_{CL}\,(L/hr)}{V_d\,(L)}$

Estimated half-life: $\dfrac{0.693}{k_e}$

Vancomycin Maintenance Dose (mg): $Cmax_{ss}$ x V_d x $(1 - e^{-keT})$

Predicted Vancomycin $Cmax_{ss}$ (mg/L): $\dfrac{Dose\,(mg)\; x\; (1 - e^{-keti})}{K_e\; x\; V_d\; x\; ti\; x\; (1 - e^{-keT})}$

Predicted Vancomycin $Cmin_{ss}$ (mg/L): $Cmax_{ss}$ x $e^{-ke(T - ti)}$

Estimated Vancomycin 24-hour Area-Under-the-Curve (mg*hr/L):
$\dfrac{Total\; vancomycin\; dose\,(mg)/24\; hours}{Vancomycin_{CL}\,(L/hr)}$

CrCl: Creatinine Clearance.
TBW: Total Body Weight.
$Vancomycin_{CL}$: Vancomycin Clearance.
V_d: Volume of Distribution.
K_e: Elimination Rate Constant.
T: Dosing Interval (hours).
ti: Infusion Time (hours).
$Cmax_{ss}$: Peak Concentration at Steady State.
$Cmin_{ss}$: Trough Concentration at Steady State.

Conclusion

Vancomycin continues to be an important antibiotic that has maintained high rates of sensitivity to *S. aureus* species. Over time, the emergence of vancomycin-intermediate *S. aureus* isolates have highlighted the importance of, not only judiciously using antibiotics like vancomycin, but ensuring they are dosed properly to optimize their pharmacokinetics and pharmacodynamics, while minimizing toxicity. The consensus recommendations on the therapeutic monitoring of vancomycin in adult patients has gone a long way to assist in standardizing how vancomycin is dosed and monitored, but evidence published since 2009 has suggested that, while important, the trough concentration may not be the only factor we should consider when dosing vancomycin. The AUC/MIC ratio continues to be very important, and could be the key to truly optimizing vancomycin dosing, while minimizing toxicity. Vancomycin dosing continues to challenge clinicians and now, it appears, the best practices in dosing should involve multiple methods, taking into account not only trough concentrations, but also the estimated vancomycin AUC and the organism MIC.

References

[1]   Levine, D. P. Vancomycin: a history. *Clin. Infect Dis.* 2006;42:S5-12.
[2]   Geraci, J. E. Vancomycin. *Mayo Clin. Proc.* 1977;52:631-4.
[3]   Ziegler, D. W.; Wolfe, R. N.; McGuire, J. M. Vancomycin, a new antibiotic.II in vitro antibacterial studies. *Antibiot Ann.* 1955;3:612-8.
[4]   Griffith, R. S.; Peck, Jr F. B. Vancomycin, a new antibiotic. III preliminary clinical and laboratory studies. *Antibiot Ann.* 1955;3:619-22.
[5]   Geraci, J. E.; Heilman, F. R.; Nichols, D. R. et al., Some laboratory and clinical experiences with a new antibiotic, vancomycin. *Mayo Clin. Proc.* 1956;31:564-82.
[6]   Craig, W. A. Basic pharmacodynamics of antibacterials with clinical applications to the use of beta-lactams, glycopeptides, and linezolid. *Infect Dis. Clin. N. Am.* 2003;17:479-501.
[7]   Ebert, S.; Leggett, J.; Vogelman, B. In vivo cidal activity and pharmacokinetics parameters (PKPs) for vancomycin against methicillin-susceptible (MSSA) and –resistant (MRSA) *S. aureus.* In: Program and abstracts of the 27th Interscience Conference on Antimicrobial Agents and Chemotherapy (New York). Washington: American Society for Microbiology; 1987:173.
[8]   Moise-Broder, P. A.; Forrest, A.; Birmingham, M. C.; Schentag, J. J. Pharmacodynamics of vancomcyin and other antimicrobials in patients with *Staphylococcus aureus* lower respiratory tract infections. *Clin. Pharmacokinet* 2004;43:925-42.
[9]   Rybak, M.; Lomaestro, B.; Rotschafer, J. C. et al., Therapeutic monitoring of vancomycin in adult patients: a consensus review of the

American Society of Health-System Pharmacists, the Infectious Diseases Society of America, and the Society of Infectious Diseases Pharmacists. *Am. J. Health-Syst. Pharm.* 2009;66:82-98.

[10] Guidelines for the management of adults with hospital-acquired, ventilator-associated, and healthcare-associated pneumonia. *Am. J. Respir. Crit. Care Med.* 2005;171:388-416.

[11] Cruciani, M.; Gatti, G.; Lazzarini, L. et al., Penetration of vancomycin into human lung tissue. *J. Antimicrob. Chemother* 1996;38:865-9.

[12] Jeffres, M. N.; Isakow, W.; Doherty, J. A. et al., Predictors of mortality for methicillin-resistant *Staphylococcus aureus* health care-associated pneumonia: specific evaluation of vancomycin pharmacokinetic indicies. *Chest* 2006;131:947-55.

[13] Kullar, R.; Davis, S. L.; Levine, D. P.; Rybak, M. J. Impact of vancomycin exposure on outcomes in patients with methicillin-resistant *Staphylococcus aureus* bacteremia: support for the consensus guidelines suggested targets. *Clin. Infect Dis.* 2011;52:975-81.

[14] Ackerman, B. H.; Guilday, R. E.; Reigart, C. L.; Patton, M. L.; Haith, L. R. Evaluation of the relationship between elevated vancomycin trough concentrations and increased efficacy and/or toxicity. *J. Burn Care Res.* 2013;34:e1-9.

[15] Kullar, R.; Davis, S. L.; Taylor, T. N.; Kaye, K. S.; Rybak, M. J. Effects of targeting higher vancomycin trough levels on clinical outcomes and costs in a matched patient cohort. *Pharmacotherapy* 2012; doi: 10.1002/PHAR.1017.

[16] Horey, A.; Mergenhagen, K. A.; Mattappallil, A. The relationship of nephrotoxicity to vancomycin trough serum concentrations in a veteran's population: a retrospective analysis. *Ann. Pharmacother* 2012;46:1477-83.

[17] Hall, R. G. 2nd; Hazlewood, K. A.; Brouse, S. D. et al., Empiric guideline-recommended weight-based vancomycin dosing and nephrotoxicity rates in patients with methicillin-reisstant Staphylococcus aureus bacteremia: a retrospective cohort study. *BMC Pharmacol. Toxicol.* 2013; 13:6511-14.

[18] Van Hal, S. J.; Paterson, D. L.; Lodise, T. P. Systematic review and meta-analysis of vancomycin-induced nephrotoxicity associated with dosing schedules that maintain troughs between 15 and 20 milligrams per liter. *Antimicrob. Agents Chemother* 2013;57:734-44.

[19] Brown, J.; Brown, K.; Forrest, A. Vancomycin AUC_{24}/MIC ratio in patients with complicated bacteremia and infective endocarditis due to

methicillin-resistant *Staphylococcus aureus* and its association with attributable mortality during hospitalization. *Antimicrob. Agents Chemother* 2012;56:634-8.

[20] Holmes, N. E.; Turnidge, J. D.; Munckhof, W. J. et al., Vancomycin AUC/MIC ratio and 30-day mortality in patients with *Staphylococcus aureus* bacteremia. *Antimcrob. Agents Chemother* 2013;57:1654-63.

[21] Le, J.; Bradley, J. S.; Murray, W. et al., Improved vancomycin dosing in children using area under the curve exposure. *Pediatr. Infect Dis. J.* 2013;32:e155-63.

[22] Patel, N.; Pai, M. P.; Rodvold, K. A. et al., Vancomycin: we can't get there from here. *Clin. Infect Dis.* 2011;52:969-74.

[23] DeRyke, C. A.; Alexander, D. P. Optimizing vancomycin dosing through pharmacodynamics assessment targeting area under the concentration-time cure/minimum inhibitory concentration. *Hosp. Pharm.* 2009;44:751-65.

In: Vancomycin   ISBN: 978-1-62948-559-1
Editor: Abu Gafar Hossion   © 2013 Nova Science Publishers, Inc.

Chapter 2

Comparative and Functional Genomics as Tools for Understanding Vancomycin Resistance in Bacteria

Andy Hesketh and *Hee-Jeon Hong**
Department of Biochemistry, University of Cambridge, UK

Abstract

Vancomycin resistance in Gram-positive bacteria can be classified as intermediate or high-level according to the differing susceptibilities that strains exhibit towards the antibiotic. Identifying the changes in genome content or expression which are associated with the acquisition of the different types of vancomycin resistance is an important step in the process of understanding the molecular basis of resistance, and has the potential to provide leads both for new drug targets and for diagnostic biomarkers. In this chapter we review the use of comparative and functional genomics approaches for addressing the questions: which adaptations in gene expression are important for determining the level of vancomycin susceptibility, and how do these produce the resultant phenotype? The picture that emerges is one where the acquisition of a

* Corresponding Co-Authors. Email: arh69@cam.ac.uk or hh309@cam.ac.uk. Mailing address: Hopkins Building, 80 Tennis Court Road, Cambridge CB2 1QW, UK.

small number of specific enzyme activities markedly reduces susceptibility, while a complex network of more generalised cellular mechanisms can be combined to produce low or intermediate effects.

Keywords: Vancomycin; resistance; genomics; staphylococcus; enterococcus

Introduction

The development and application of antibiotic therapies in the 20th century revolutionised the treatment of bacterial infections, but early hopes of a final solution to the suffering caused by human pathogens were soon put into perspective by the rapid appearance of resistance (see Levy and Marshall [1], and Davies and Davies [2] for recent interesting reviews). During the 1950s and 1960s the emergence of resistant pathogens seemed however to be of only minor concern as new antibiotics with novel mechanisms of action were continually being discovered to combat the resistant strains. Vancomycin, a natural metabolite first isolated from *Amycolotopsis orientalis*, was one such compound [3]. Approved for use in 1958, it exhibited the unusual activity of inhibiting an essential step in bacterial cell wall biosynthesis not via interaction with the enzyme, but by sequestering the substrate used by the enzyme [4] (Figure 1). Today however we live in a world where resistance has emerged for all the antibiotics in clinical use, and where the discovery pipeline for generating replacement therapies has dwindled down to a small fraction of its former self [5].

A future scenario where no effective treatments exist for common bacterial infections is therefore increasingly being seen as a real possibility, and the global spread of resistant pathogens, and resistance genes, is being closely monitored (e.g. http://www.cdc.gov/narms/; http://www.crl-ar.eu/; http://www.who.int/drugresistance/surveillance/en/). Vancomycin resistance in bacterial pathogens first emerged in enterococci in the 1980s, followed over a decade later by resistance in *Staphylococcus aureus* (Figure 2; reviewed in [6]). Vancomycin resistant eneterococci (VRE) typically exhibit a high level of resistance to the antibiotic with a minimum inhibitory concentration (MIC) of 16 µg/ml or higher when cultivated in liquid culture, and have been classified into sub-types according to the genes encoding the resistance activity (Figure 2b). Highly resistant strains of *S. aureus* (VRSA) have also been isolated, but intermediate resistance strains (VISA; MIC = 4-8 µg/ml) and heterogeneous-intermediate (hVISA; a mixed population of vancomycin susceptible (MIC <2 µg/ml) and intermediately resistant cells) are more common. Understanding the processes by which antibiotics come to fail to be effective will have an important role to play in the formulation of future strategies for counteracting the worsening problems with resistance and preventing an unwelcome return to the treatments employed in the days before antibiotics were first discovered. This includes both a detailed knowledge of the changes occurring in the bacterial genome which give the potential for a reduced susceptibility towards a particular antibiotic, and an integrated understanding of how the altered genotype produces the troublesome end result. Such information has the potential to identify new cellular targets for the development of novel antibacterial therapies, to inform the rational design of modified activities, and to suggest opportunities for synergistically combining the effects of different antibacterial compounds to increase their overall potency.

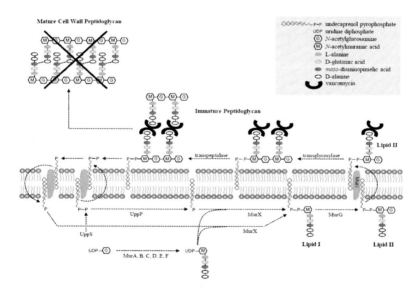

Figure 1. Model illustrating bacterial cell wall peptidoglycan biosynthesis and the mode of action of vancomycin. Based on studies in *Escherichia coli*, lipid II complete with its pentapeptide side chain is assembled in the cytoplasm before being transported through the membrane and polymerised by transglycosylase to form immature peptidoglycan. Introduction of cross-links by the action of the transpeptidase enzyme then forms mature peptidoglycan. Vancomycin binds to the D-Ala-D-Ala dipeptide termini of non-cross-linked peptidoglycan pentapeptide side chains preventing the formation of mature peptidoglycan and lowering the strength and rigidity of the cell wall. This renders the bacteria susceptible to osmotic lysis.

A

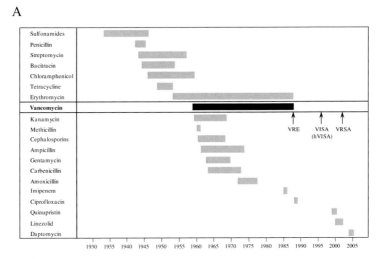

B

Phenotype	Mechanism of Resistance	Resistance to	Induction
VRE-VanA	Reprograming of PG precursors from D-Ala-D-Ala to D-Ala-D-Lac via VanHAX	vancomycin, teicoplanin	inducible
VRE-VanB	Reprograming of PG precursors from D-Ala-D-Ala to D-Ala-D-Lac via VanHAX	vancomycin	inducible
VRE-VanC	Reprograming of PG precursors from D-Ala-D-Ala to D-Ala-D-Ser via VanHAX	vancomycin	inducible, constitutive
VRE-VanD	Reprograming of PG precursors from D-Ala-D-Ala to D-Ala-D-Lac via VanHAX	vancomycin, teicoplanin	constitutive
VRE-VanE	Reprograming of PG precursors from D-Ala-D-Ala to D-Ala-D-Ser via VanHAX	vancomycin	inducible
VRE-VanG	Reprograming of PG precursors from D-Ala-D-Ala to D-Ala-D-Ser via VanHAX	vancomycin	inducible
VRSA-VanA	Reprograming of PG precursors from D-Ala-D-Ala to D-Ala-D-Lac via VanHAX	vancomycin, teicoplanin	inducible
VISA (hVISA)	Thickening of the cell wall via multiple loci	vancomycin, teicoplanin	constitutive

Figure 2. A) The emergence of antibiotic resistance (end of bar) in pathogenic bacteria, viewed in the context of their date of first use in the clinic (beginning of bar). VRE= vancomycin resistant enterococci; VISA/hVISA = intermediate/heterogeneous-intermediate resistant *Staphylococcus aureus*; VRSA = vancomycin resistant *S. aureus*. B) Classification of resistant enterococcal and staphylococcal strains into sub-types according to the mechanism of resistance.

Fortunately, recent technological advances in DNA sequencing have driven a huge explosion in the production of genome sequence data, as illustrated by the submission of the 1000th prokaryotic genome to databases in 2010 [7]. This increase in availability has in turn facilitated an expansion in the related sciences of comparative and functional genomics. Comparative genomics aims to identify the differences in genotype that are important for the expression of a particular phenotypic trait, while functional genomics seeks to understand the mechanisms behind the causal relationship between genome and phenotype. Comparative genomics approaches are perhaps most familiar in the field of human biology where sequence data from diseased and healthy individuals are compared in order to drill down to the changes in the genetic landscape that are driving the disease state [8,9]. While they are also used extensively to study other traits in complex eukaryotes - cereal crop resistance and improvement [10], livestock breeding [11,12] - they are perhaps most powerfully applicable to the analysis of microbial genomes where the relatively small genome size (typically between 2 and 12 Mbp) puts the sequencing of a large number of similar strains within easy reach [13]. In the following sections we will review the use of comparative genomics approaches for understanding the acquisition and spread of vancomycin resistance among bacterial populations, and will take a critical look at the contribution that functional genomics analysis is making towards dissecting the cellular mechanisms that are important for conferring reduced vancomycin susceptibility. We do not intend to suggest that these techniques are by themselves sufficient to understand vancomycin resistance, but do wish to highlight the useful role they can play in this process when used alongside more traditional biochemical and molecular genetic approaches.

Comparative Genomics and Vancomycin Resistance

Comparative genomics in the context of antibiotic resistance hit the headlines in the UK in 2012 when information gleaned from sequencing isolates of meticillin-resistant *Staphylococcus aureus* (MRSA) during an infectious outbreak in a special care baby unit at a hospital in Cambridge was credited with helping to put an end to its spread (http://www.bbc.co.uk/news/health-20314024).

In their report of the incident the researchers, led by Professor Sharon Peacock, describe how the whole-genome sequencing of 12 strains isolated from the different infants who became infected in the unit over a six month period allowed a common source for the outbreak to be identified and subsequently tracked down to an asymptomatic carrier working on the ward as a member of the staff [14]. The success of the study suggested that such a genome sequencing approach could be a rapid and cost-effective way to accurately identify pathways of bacterial transmission in hospital and community settings, ultimately enabling reductions in infections and morbidity. Prior to this report however, comparative genomics analysis of *S. aureus* was already being commonly applied in research laboratories across the world, primarily to understand the processes involved in the evolution of pathogenic and meticillin resistant strains [15-18]. In contrast to meticillin, the use of vancomycin in the clinic has been consciously restricted and it is typically reserved as a last line of defence treatment for serious infections that exhibit resistance to the more commonly used antibiotics e.g. MRSA. Bacterial resistance to vancomycin is consequently much rarer than that seen towards meticillin, and there have thus far been fewer comparative genomics studies reported.

Table 1 summarises the literature reporting investigations into the genomic basis of vancomycin resistance, and these will be considered in more detail in the following sections subdivided according to the identity of the resistant species under investigation.

I) *Staphylococcus aureus*

Kuroda *et al.* reported the first comparative study concerning vancomycin resistance in the Lancet in 2001 using *S. aureus* strains isolated from patients in a Japanese hospital [19]. The genome of the first clinically isolated vancomycin resistant MRSA strain Mu50 [20] was sequenced and compared to the vancomycin-susceptible MRSA strain N315 [21]. Mu50 does not possess the inducible *vanA* or *vanB* resistance genes associated with high-level vancomycin resistance, but exhibits an intermediate level resistance that is characterised by cell wall thickening and changes in cell wall composition and turnover [22-24]. The shotgun DNA sequencing approach used in this early analysis was considerably more expensive and time-consuming than the methods now available, and the study consequently suffered from the effect of the small number of strains analysed undermining the certainty with which observed changes in genotype could be causally linked to the phenotypes of interest. This problem was exacerbated by the fact that the two strains being compared, although isolated from patients in the same hospital in Tokyo, were not closely matched with one another. N315 was isolated in 1982 and Mu50 in 1997.

Table 1. Comparative genomics studies of vancomycin resistant bacteria

Organism	Summary of the study	Ref.
Staphylococcus aureus	Comparison of the first clinical (intermediate-level) vancomycin resistant MRSA strain Mu50 with a vancomycin susceptible MRSA strain N315.	[19]
Staphylococcus aureus	Comparison of the first clinical vancomycin resistant MRSA strain Mu50 with the vancomycin susceptible MRSA strains N315, EMRSA16, and COL.	[25]
Enterococcus faecalis	Sequencing of first vancomycin resistant clinical isolate of *E. faecalis* in the United States, strain V583, and comparison with sections of the genomes of other pathogenic isolates MMH594 and V586.	[46, 47]
Staphylococcus aureus	A re-evaluation of the comparison of N315 and Mu50 by the original authors, including some sequence analysis of a third clinical strain exhibiting low level vancomycin resistance Mu3.	[26]
Staphylococcus aureus	Comparison of an isogenic matched pair of MRSA strains isolated from the same patient before and after treatment with vancomycin. The initial strain was fully susceptible to vancomycin, while the final strain exhibited intermediate resistance (8 μg/ml).	[31]
Staphylococcus aureus	Comparison of an isogenic matched pair of MRSA strains isolated from the same patient before and after 42 days of treatment with vancomycin. The initial strain was fully susceptible to vancomycin, while the final strain exhibited intermediate resistance (4 μg/ml).	[32]
Staphylococcus aureus	Comparison of a fully vancomycin susceptible MRSA strain (N315) with related strains exhibiting heterogeneous intermediate (Mu3) and intermediate (Mu50) vancomycin resistance.	[35]
Staphylococcus aureus	Comparison of a fully vancomycin susceptible strain (Mu50Ω) with a related strain Mu50 exhibiting intermediate resistance (not a clinical matched pair).	[34]
Enterococcus faecium	Sequencing of two different high-level vancomycin resistant strains isolated from a clinical setting.	[52]
Enterococcus faecium	Comparison of five strains isolated from hospitalised patients, two of which exhibited high-level VanA-type vancomycin resistance, with two isolated from healthy non-hospitalised individuals.	[51]
Staphylococcus aureus	Sequencing of 10 strains to analyse the genetic basis of vancomycin intermediate and heterogeneous-vancomycin intermediate resistance. Five isogenic matched pairs of clinical strains from patients who failed vancomycin therapy, including reanalysis of a pair first reported in [32].	[33]
Staphylococcus aureus	Sequencing of 14 strains to analyse the genetic basis of vancomycin intermediate resistance. Three isogenic matched pairs of clinical strains from patients who failed vancomycin therapy; a series of five clinical strains isolated from a patient during a similar failed treatment; and a series of three strains produced in the laboratory by vancomycin passage.	[36]
Staphylococcus aureus	Analysis of the strains from all 12 cases of VRSA (high-level vancomycin resistance) identified in the United States from 2002-2012.	[37]
Actinomycetes	Contains a comparison of vancomycin resistance gene homologues in six streptomycete genomes, a group of ubiquitous soil dwelling bacteria that produce many of the world's antibiotics.	[61]

Table 1. (Continued)

Organism	Summary of the study	Ref.
Enterococcus sp.	Comparative analysis of 28 genome sequences from *E. faecalis, E. faecium, E. casseliflavus* and *E. gallinarum*. Includes clinical isolates, commensal strains and vancomycin resistant strains.	[49, 54, 55]
Enterococcus faecalis	A comparative analysis involving 63 strains based on publically available genome sequences.	[53]
Enterococcus faecium	The first complete *E. faecium* genome sequence, of a clinical high-level vancomycin resistant isolate.	[48]
Enterococcus faecium	A comparison of the genomes of 22 sequenced strains, including six exhibiting high-level VanA-type resistance.	[50]
Staphylococcus aureus	A comparison of two USA300 MRSA isolates collected sequentially from a single patient; a vancomycin susceptible strain A1-VSSA, and an intermediate resistant strain A2-VISA (MIC 8 µg/ml).	[38]

Despite these limitations the analysis was a landmark in providing both the first reference genome sequences for *S. aureus,* and an early global insight into the importance of lateral gene transfer events and mobile genetic elements in the biology of *S. aureus.* The nucleotide sequence identity between the two strains was found to be 96%, with most of the differences being due to mobile genetic elements acquired by the Mu50 genome. These included a 25 Kbp plasmid pMU50 carrying resistance determinants for aminoglycoside antibiotics and quaternary ammonium compounds. Both strains carried an integrated copy of the staphylococcal cassette chromosome *mec* (SSCmec) encoding resistance towards meticillin and a number of other antibiotics (bleomycin, spectinomycin, aminoglycosides, macrolides), and also three previously unidentified pathogenicity islands. However, despite identifying a catalogue of approximately 70 new *S. aureus* virulence factor candidate genes the report of the comparison failed to directly address the question of the difference in vancomycin resistance between the two strains. This important issue was picked up on in two subsequent papers which reanalysed the original sequences together with additional MRSA genome sequence data [25, 26] (Table 2). Avison *et al.* [25] included the genome sequences of the COL and EMRSA-16 vancomycin-susceptible MRSA strains which had been made publicly available through the Sanger and TIGR sequencing centres, respectively. They identified 164 mutagenic sequence changes in the ORFs shared by the N315 and Mu50 strains, 114 leading to single amino acid substitutions and 50 producing deletions, frame-shift mutations or truncations in the Mu50 proteins. Of the latter loss of function changes, 37 were also conserved in comparison with both the COL or EMRSA-16 strains indicating a possible causal link with the vancomycin resistance phenotype.

Table 2. Summary of the major findings from comparative genomics analysis of the evolution of vancomycin resistance in *S. aureus* referred to in Table 1

Ref.	Mutations identified and considered in association with vancomycin resistance
[19, 25, 26]	• Mutagenic changes in ca. 200 loci • Missense point mutation in the VraS sensor kinase • Missense point mutations in the alternative sigma factors SigA and SigB • Loss of function mutations in biosynthetic enzymes putatively influencing peptidogycan synthesis
[31]	• Missense point mutations in 31 loci • Point mutation in SA1702, a protein from the same operon as *vraR* • Point mutation in SA1249, a protein of unknown function • Frameshift mutation in AgrC from the *agr* quorum sensing locus • Truncation of YycH putatively involved in the regulation of a cell wall lyticase
[32]	• Missense point mutations in 6 loci • Point mutation in the GraS sensor kinase
[35]	• Missense point mutations in 9 loci between a heterogeneous intermediate and intermediate resistance strain • Point mutation in the GraR response regulator
[34]	• Mutagenic changes in 13 loci • Missense point mutation in the GraR response regulator • Missense mutation leading to truncation of the VraS sensor kinase
[33]	• Mutation in the *walKR* locus in four out of five cases where matched pairs of susceptible and nonsuceptible clinical isolates were compared
[36]	• Mutagenic changes in a total of 30 loci when comparing 4 matched pairs of susceptible and nonsuceptible clinical isolates • Very little overlap in the changes between each pair – only RpsU shared between two pairs • Point mutation in SA1702, a protein originating from the same operon as *vraR* • Acquisition of a mutation in WalK during laboratory selection for vancomycin resistance • Identification and experimental confirmation of the importance of a mutation in the serine/threonine phosphatase Stp1
[37]	• High-level vancomycin resistance associated with the acquisition of transposon Tn1546 (putatively from enterococcal donors) in all 12 cases of clinical VRSA analysed • All 12 acquisition events believed to have occurred independently from one another • No mutations identified in restriction barrier systems • Loss of function mutation in DprA in 11/12 strains
[38]	• 6 insertion/deletion events identified between the susceptible and resistant strains analysed • The significance of a 6 bp nonframeshift insertion into a metal binding motif in the serine/threonine phosphatase *stp1* was characterised experimentally • Comparison with laboratory evolution of resistance in the susceptible isolate suggests multiple routes towards vancomycin non-susceptibility.

While many were in proteins with no known function, the authors interpreted five of the mutations observed in biosynthetic enzymes as potentially playing a role in the known changes in peptidoglycan biosynthesis in Mu50. The mutations in coding sequence leading to single amino acid changes were not however considered, a significant omission in light of the results of more recent studies. Meanwhile, the authors of the original paper responded with their own reinterpretation, including in their analysis a second intermediate vancomycin resistant isolate Mu3 [26]. Mu3 was not sequenced in its entirety, the focus instead being placed on only those regions highlighted as being different between Mu50 and N315 in order to determine the conserved changes that may be linked to the vancomycin resistance phenotype. In this way Mu50 and Mu3 were found to possess 204 sequence changes in common (49 predicted to produce loss of function changes) which were concentrated in three major functional categories; sugar transport, glutamate metabolism and transcriptional regulation. Changes in cell wall peptidoglycan biosynthesis in the vancomycin resistant strains were attributed to the putative changes in sugar transport and glutamate biosynthesis, and it was speculated that observed point mutations in the alternative sigma factors SigA and SigB, and in the VraS sensor kinase may indicate a signalling role for these proteins in the adaptation of *S. aureus* to the presence of vancomycin. While no attempts were made to confirm any of the hypotheses generated in either publication, recent molecular genetic studies have confirmed an important role for VraS and its partner two-component regulator VraR in coordinating a response to cell wall damage [27,28]. Point mutations in the *vraSR* genes have also been implicated in the evolution of vancomcyin resistant strains in the clinic in many of the comparative genomics studies which were to follow (see below and Table 2). Interestingly, a role for the alternative sigma factor SigA in the regulation of VraS expression has been reported [29], while SigB has been shown to coordinate a response to a variety of environmental stresses in *S. aureus* [30]. Functional genomics studies using strains engineered with mutations in some of these genes have been used to further define their role in adaptation to vancomycin (see below).

While the first comparative genomics analyses of vancomycin resistance in *S. aureus* described above produced some interesting observations, some of which turned out to be of genuine significance, the studies were hampered by the small number of strains sequenced and by the absence of specific before-and-after-treatment matching of the clinical isolates analysed. The major contribution of these initial studies was probably therefore in creating the reference genome sequences and providing genome-wide information about potential virulence factors and pathogenicity islands. Pulsed-field gel electrophoresis (PFGE) and multilocus sequence typing (MLST) provided cheaper, more readily accessible ways of assessing genomic variability between clinical isolates exhibiting antibiotic resistance, albeit at a much lower level of resolution. However, the proof of principle had been established and as the well-documented improvements in DNA sequencing methods started to produce significant reductions in the costs and time required for sequencing a genome, comparative studies were resumed using both larger numbers of strains and, importantly, matched pairs of strains isolated from the same patient before and after a failed vancomycin treatment [31-38]. The major findings from these studies is summarised in Table 2. The group led by Alexander Tomasz set the standard for experimental design in their elegant studies of the *in vivo* evolution of antibiotic resistance in isogenic *S. aureus* isolates recovered periodically from the bloodstream of a patient undergoing chemotherapy with rifampin, imipenem and vancomycin [39-41]. Nine samples were taken over the course of a 12 week period of treatment (which ultimately ended in the patient's death) during which rifampin was soon identified as having become ineffective and replaced by a combination of imipenem and vancomycin. Whole genome sequencing of the first vancomycin susceptible isolate (MIC = 1 μg/ml) and last non-susceptible isolate (MIC = 8 μg/ml) identified the acquisition of only 35 point mutations in just 31 loci [40]. The presence of these mutations in the intermediate samples isolated was analysed by targeted sequencing and revealed a sequential accumulation of increasing numbers of the mutations as the therapy progressed, the key events being identified as the early appearance of mutations leading to four amino acid changes in the β-subunit of RNA polymerase which likely specify the resistance to rifampin; a point mutation reversing a pre-existing frameshift mutation in *blaR1* which restores β-lactam resistance; and the sequential acquisition of mutations in a protein associated with the VraR regulator, a protein AgrC from the *agr* quorum sensing locus, and a truncation of YycH, all of which correlate with the appearance of increasing resistance to vancomycin. Interestingly, a targeted PCR sequencing analysis of the *vraR* operon in seven geographically diverse intermediate vancomycin resistant isolates of *S. aureus,* including the archetypal vancomycin resistance strain Mu50, identified mutations in all seven, consistent with an important role for these genes in the sequential acquisition of resistance. In contrast to this study however, Cameron *et al.* [36] observed a loss of some mutations acquired during the evolution of vancomycin resistance in their analysis of a different time series of matched clinical isolates, and in addition identified only one repeated gene mutation out of a total of 30 found in a comparison of four matched pairs of susceptible/nonsusceptible clinical strains. This highlighted a heterogeneity in both the population of strains present and in the genetic changes associated with exposure to vancomycin in a clinical setting, and suggests that there are likely to be many routes to the *in vivo* acquisition of intermediate level resistance to the antibiotic. Focusing on one of the novel changes observed, a point mutation causing truncation of the serine/threonine phosphatase Stp1, the authors did nonetheless demonstrate that their comparative approach was capable of yielding biologically relevant gene candidates. Engineered deletion of *stp1* in a vancomycin susceptible strain increased its resistance to the antibiotic into the nonsusceptible range, a change which could be reversed by complementation with a functional copy of the gene.

The MIC of the engineered *stp1* mutant strain was noticeably lower than for the nonsusceptible clinical isolate however, 3 µg/ml compared with 4 µg/ml, suggesting some auxiliary effect of the other mutations identified in the clinical isolate. Mutation of *stp1* was identified as being associated with the evolution of vancomycin resistance in a study analyzing USA300 MRSA isolates collected from a patient with endocarditis [38]. Only six differences were identified between the susceptible (MIC = 1 µg/ml) and non-susceptible (MIC = 8 µg/ml) strains analysed, and the significance of a 6 bp insertion into *stp1* in the non-susceptible strain was experimentally demonstrated when complementation with a wild-type copy of the gene partially restored the vancomycin susceptibility phenotype (MIC = 4 µg/ml). Molecular genetic experiments have also been used to investigate the role of mutations in the *vraSR*, *graSR*, and *walKR* two-component signal transduction systems which have been identified in several of the comparative genomics studies [32-35]. Howden *et al.* [33] conducted bi-directional allelic exchange experiments between their susceptible/nonsusceptible pairs of clinical strains and showed that single nucleotide substitutions within either *walK* or *walR* led to vancomycin resistance and caused the typical cell wall thickening observed in resistant clinical isolates. Similarly, introduction of a mutated copy of the *graR* regulatory gene (but not a wild-type copy) was found to be sufficient to convert the strain Mu3 exhibiting heterogenous-intermediate resistance into a fully intermediate resistant strain with a phenotype comparable to Mu50 [35]. The significance of the same amino acid substitution in GraR was confirmed in an analogous experiment using a different nonsusceptible host background strain Mu50Ω [34], and the engineering of a mutation in *graS* has also been shown to confer an increase in resistance to vancomycin in a previously susceptible clinical isolate [32]. Genetic manipulation of the vancomycin susceptible Mu50Ω strain also verified the importance of mutations detected in *vraS* for conferring resistance to the antibiotic, and a double change in *vraS* and *graR* yielded a strain comparable to Mu50 [34].

Only one comparative genomics study has been reported on high-level resistance to vancomycin in *S. aureus* (VRSA), presumably because MLST is sufficient to identify lateral acquisition of the dedicated *van* resistance genes whose expression is induced to enable them to cope with the higher concentrations of the antibiotic. Kos *et al.* [37] sequenced twelve clonal cluster 5 (CC5) VRSA strains isolated from all the clinical cases that occurred in the United States between 2002 and 2012. Their analysis confirmed that in all cases the resistance was attributable to acquisition of a *vanA* resistance gene carried on a Tn1564 transposable element and presumably of enterococcal origin. Interestingly however, the availability of the whole genome sequences for each strain allowed them to investigate whether the strains were derived from shared transposition events, and whether or not the CC5 genotype may predispose or otherwise enhance the ability of *S. aureus* to acquire and express transposable vancomycin resistance. The latter question is particularly significant since CC5 lineage strains are the leading causes of hospital-associated MRSA infections in the United States [42]. From the sequence analysis the authors were able to conclude that, although the isolates clustered according to the geographical location of their occurrence, each transposon acquisition event had happened independently from one another, consistent with the hypothesis that the strains underwent transposition during the course of the infection. No evidence for a weakening in the *S. aureus* restriction barrier system was detected, but eleven out of the twelve strains possessed a loss of function mutation in the *dprA* gene which plays a poorly defined role in DNA transformation efficiency in naturally competent bacteria, thus suggesting a potentially interesting candidate target gene for future study.

II) *Enterococcus faecalis* and *Enterococcus faecium*

Enterococci form part of the natural microflorae of the digestive tracts of humans, other mammals, insects and birds. They are Gram-positive lactic acid bacteria which have also found use in probiotic formulations and food production. In recent years however, *E. faecalis* and *E. faecium*, the two species most commonly associated with human gastrointestinal tract colonization, have emerged as leading causes of multidrug resistant hospital acquired infections of the urinary tract, heart and surgical wounds (for a review see [43]). The mechanisms by which these well adapted symbiotic bacteria have evolved into hospital pathogens are still only partly understood, but their appearance has correlated with the increasing use of antibiotic therapies. Indeed, the emergence of hospital-associated enterococcal infections in the United States has been described as taking place in two distinct waves: the first beginning in the 1970s, dominated by *E. faecalis* strains and associated with the introduction of third-generation cephalosporins; followed by a second wave starting in the 1990s involving a steady increase in drug resistant *E. faecium* infections, and associated with the increasing use of vancomycin [44, 45]. Interestingly during this period the proportion of vancomycin resistant *E. faecalis* clinical isolates was consistently around 5%, while in contrast *E. faecium* showed a dramatic increase from 0% in the mid-1980s to ca. 80% by 2007. Vancomycin resistance in enterococci is typically high-level resistance associated with the inducible expression of dedicated *vanA* or *vanB* type genes originating from horizontal gene transfer events, and PFGE and MLST have proven to be effective tools for serotyping clinical isolates, and tracking the acquisition of the drug resistance genes. However, since 2002 whole-genome sequencing approaches have increasingly been used to compare different pathogenic and non-pathogenic enterococcal strains in attempts to identify virulence factors and to understand differences in the acquisition of drug resistance determinants (see Table 1).

The first enterococcal genome sequence reported was of the first vancomycin resistant clinical isolate of *E. faecalis* in the United States, strain V583 [46]. Analysis of the sequence suggested that a surprisingly high proportion of the genome, ca. 25%, consists of probable mobile or foreign DNA, including a *vanB* vancomycin-resistance conjugative transposon. Shankar *et al.* [47] compared elements of the V583 sequence with those from a vancomycin susceptible *E. faecalis* clinical isolate MMH594, but their focus was on identification of a common 153 Kbp pathogenicity island and factors surrounding the acquisition of the vancomycin resistance genetic element were not explored. The first complete *E. faecium* genome sequence did not arrive on the scene until 2012 [48], but in the intervening period the draft genome sequences of many 10s of different enterococcal strains were determined and analysed [49-55]. The major driving force behind these comparative studies was to more fully understand the versatility of enterococci in colonizing a diverse range of environments and hosts, and their success as opportunistic pathogens (see Santagati *et al.* [56] for a useful review). Although this is still far from being fully explained, the studies have reinforced the initial observations concerning the importance of mobile genetic elements for their remarkable adaptability. Indeed, in a comparison of the genomes of seven strains, van Schaik *et al.* concluded that the *E. faecium* pan-genome is essentially unlimited, and that hospital-associated isolates accumulate genomic elements related to antibiotic resistance and colonization [51]. Comparative analysis involving 16 *E. faecalis* strains reached a similar conclusion, and identified a strong inverse correlation between CRISPR (clustered regularly interspaced short palindromic repeats) loci and acquired antibiotic resistance [44,54,55]. CRIPSR loci are widespread in prokaryotes where they are known to confer resistance to plasmid and phage entry, and their absence in the antibiotic resistant *E. faecalis* isolates suggests that exposure to antibiotics inadvertently selects for strains lacking this defence mechanism and thus is likely to promote the acquisition of mobile DNA. Interestingly, the seven *E. faecium* strains discussed above were also found to lack CRIPSR [51], and in an analysis of a further eight additional strains, including four which lack acquired antibiotic resistance genes, CRIPSR loci were identified in three strains, but were strikingly absent from all vancomycin resistant isolates tested [55]. However, in their analysis of 21 *E. faecium* genomes (including those already mentioned above) Qin *et al.* [50] identified only a total of four which contained the CRISPR locus, one of which also possessed antibiotic resistance associated genes. The inverse relationship between the presence of CRISPR and antibiotic resistance determinants does not therefore always hold true, and the authors noted a requirement for more *E. faecium* strains containing CRISPR loci to be sequenced to clarify the significance of this relationship.

III) Actinomycetes

In addition to pathogenic species such as *S. aureus*, *E. faecalis* and *E. faecium*, inducible high-level resistance to vancomycin also occurs in harmless free-living bacteria, most notably soil-dwelling actinomycetes and *Paenibacillus* species. *Paenibacillus thiaminolyticus* and *Paenibacillus apiaries* both contain functional vancomycin resistance gene clusters homologous to those found in hospital-associated enterococcal species, and it has been proposed that the *van* operons in the two organisms have evolved from a common ancestor [57]. Another perhaps more plausible source for the origin of vancomycin resistance genes is the group of organisms which produce glycopeptide antibiotics as natural secondary metabolites, the actinomycetes. Actinomycete species, including *Nonomurea, Amycolotopsis, Actinoplanes* and *Streptomyces*, in addition to carrying the genes which direct the synthesis and export of the glycopeptides, also contain genes for self-resistance to the compounds they produce. Since they are naturally paired with the biosynthesis of a known glycopeptide structure, the resistance gene clusters in these producing organisms have been of particular interest for investigating the specificity of the signalling systems which sense and coordinate the response to the presence of the antibiotic [58-60]. This is typically mediated via a two-component signal transduction system consisting of a VanS sensor kinase and a cognate VanR response regulator, the latter ultimately being responsible for up-regulation of the transcription of all the genes in the resistance cluster. Although a recent search of the GOLD Genomes Online Database (http://www.genomesonline.org; April 2013) revealed 140 draft or complete genome sequences for *Streptomyces* species, 83 for *Paenibacillus* species and 23 for *Amycolatopsis* species, only a very limited comparative analysis of glycopeptide resistance genes in these strains could be found in the literature. Novotna *et al.* [61] analysed the distribution of homologues to the *vanJ* gene from the *Streptomyces coelicolor* vancomycin resistance cluster, and identified five other streptomycete strains where an orthologue of *vanJ* was located on the chromosome adjacent to *vanRS* and/or *vanHAX* vancomcyin resistance gene determinants. One of the strains, *S. toyocaensis*, is the producing organism of the A47934 glycopeptide, but the implication that all the strains identified also possess some form of inducible resistance to glycopeptide antibiotics is yet to be tested.

Functional Genomics and Vancomycin Resistance

Identifying the genetic changes linked to the acquisition of vancomycin resistant phenotypes by techniques such as comparative genomics can only take us part of the way towards understanding the mechanisms of resistance in bacterial populations. For a more complete picture it is also desirable to determine how the observed changes alter gene expression to effect the increased antibiotic resistance, and to analyse how bacteria respond and adapt to the presence of vancomycin in their environment. Table 3 lists the global expression studies, from both transcriptome and proteome analysis pipelines, which have focused on some aspect of vancomycin resistance or activity over the last 13 years. These will be considered in the four following categories.

Table 3. Functional genomics studies analysing vancomycin activity and resistance

Analysis	Organism	Summary	Ref.
i) Analysis of the evolution of vancomycin resistance			
Transcriptome	*Staphylococcus aureus*	Comparison of the transcriptomes of three MRSA strains exhibiting vancomycin susceptible (MU50Ω), heterogenous-intermediate resistance (MU3), and intermediate resistance (MU50) phenotypes.	[62]
Transcriptome	*Streptococcus pneumoniae*	Transcriptome analysis comparing the response to vancomycin in susceptible and resistant strains.	[64]
Transcriptome	*Staphylococcus aureus*	Comparison of the transcriptomes of a matched pair of clinical isolates exhibiting vancomycin susceptible (JH1), and intermediate resistance (JH9) phenotypes. Includes a comparison of the global response to vancomycin for each strain.	[39]
Proteome	*Staphylococcus aureus*	Three isogenic strains exhibiting different vancomycin susceptibilities and derived from a clinical vancomycin-intermediate isolate were examined by comparative protein abundance analysis.	[65]
Proteome &Transcriptome	*Staphylococcus aureus*	To unravel molecular targets involved in glycopeptide antibiotic resistance, three isogenic strains of *S. aureus* with different susceptibility levels to vancomycin or teicoplanin were subjected to whole-genome microarray based transcription and quantitative proteomic profiling.	[63]
Proteome	*Staphylococcus aureus*	Proteome profiling of proteins present in the cell envelope of intermediate level vancomycin resistance strains HIP5827 and VP32.	[66]
Proteome	*Staphylococcus aureus*	A proteomic comparison of clinical MRSA and intermediate vancomycin resistant strains.	[67]
Transcriptome	*Staphylococcus aureus*	Comparative transcriptome study of vancomycin susceptible strains with those exhibiting heterogenous-intermediate and intermediate resistance to elucidate the mechanisms underlying the changes in resistance.	[68]
Proteome	*Enterococcus faecalis*	Comparative proteomics analysis of the response to vancomycin in a clinical isolate exhibiting VanA-type resistance (V309) with the VanB-type resistance reference strain V583.	[69]
Proteome	*Enterococcus faecalis Staphylococus aureus*	Proteomics study using photoaffinity labelled vancomycin derivatives. Vancomycin susceptible and resistant strains of both *S. aureus* and *E. faecalis* were analysed to identify cellular protein targets of vancomycin.	[70]

Table 3. (Continued)

Analysis	Organism	Summary	Ref.
Transcriptome	*Staphylococcus aureus*	RNA-seq transcriptome analysis of a matched pair of clinical isolates obtained from the same patient where the first isolate was vancomycin susceptible and the second exhibited intermediate resistance.	[38]
ii) Construction and analysis of engineered mutations to define their role in resistance			
Transcriptome	*Staphylococcus aureus*	Transcriptome analysis of a *vraSR* two-component system deletion mutant strain to characterise its role in the response to vancomycin treatment.	[72]
Proteome	*Listeria monocytogenes*	Proteome analysis of a *sigB* sigma factor deletion mutant strain to characterise its role in the response to vancomycin treatment.	[73]
Transcriptome	*Bacillus subtilis*	Transcriptome analysis of a *sigM* ECF sigma factor deletion mutant strain to characterise its role in the response to vancomycin treatment.	[74]
Transcriptome (also see Table 1)	*Staphylococcus aureus*	Transcriptome analysis of a serine/threonine phosphatase *stp1* deletion mutant strain to characterise the basis of its reduced susceptibility to vancomycin.	[36]
Transcriptome (also see Table 1)	*Staphylococcus aureus*	Global transcriptome analysis to characterise the effects of point mutations in the *walK* and *walR* regulatory genes which are associated with reduced susceptibility to vancomycin and daptomycin in clinical isolates.	[33]
iii) Characterisation of the changes in gene expression induced by vancomycin treatment			
Transcriptome	*Bacillus subtilis*	Global transcriptional signature of the response to vancomycin.	[76]
Proteome	*Bacillus subtilis*	Proteomic signatures of the response to 30 different antibiotics, including vancomycin.	[75]
Transcriptome	*Bacillus licheniformis*	Global transcriptional signatures of the response to bacitracin and vancomycin.	[80]
Transcriptome	*Bacillus subtilis*	Global transcriptional signatures of the response to 37 antibiotics, including vancomycin.	[77]
Transcriptome	*Bacillus subtilis*	Transcriptional signatures of the response to 16 different antibiotics, including vancomycin.	[78]
Transcriptome	*Staphylococcus aureus*	Characterisation of the global transcriptomic response to vancomycin in the meticillin-susceptible strain Newman.	[79]
Transcriptome	*Staphylococcus aureus*	Comparison of the global transcriptional response to treatment with vancomycin, daptomycin, nisin and carbonyl cyanide m-chlorophenylhydrazone (CCCP). To characterise the mode of action of the lipopeptide antibiotic daptomycin.	[81]
Transcriptome	*Mycobacterium tuberculosis*	Characterisation of the transcriptional response induced in *M. tuberculosis* following exposure to inhibitory or sub-inhibitory concentrations of vancomycin.	[84]

Analysis	Organism	Summary	Ref.
Transcriptome	*Streptomyces coelicolor*	Transcriptional signatures of the response to treatment with vancomycin, bacitracin and moenomycin; three antibiotics which target distinct stages of cell wall biosynthesis.	[82]
Transcriptome	*Staphylococcus aureus*	Transcriptional signatures of the response to treatment with vancomycin, telavancin, enduracidin and carbonyl cyanide m-chlorophenylhydrazone (CCCP). To characterise the mode of action of the semi-synthetic vancomycin derivative telavancin.	[83]
iv) Miscellaneous studies on other aspects of vancomycin resistance and activity			
Proteome &Transcriptome	*Enterococcus faecalis*	Characterisation of the response of a vancomycin resistant strain V583 to bile acid stress.	[87, 88]
Proteome	*Enterococcus sp.*	Proteome analysis of two VanA-type vancomycin resistant isolates recovered from seagull faecal samples.	[90]
Metabolome	*Mus musculus*	Metabolomics analysis of urine and faecal samples taken from mice treated with vancomycin.	[86]
Transcriptome	*Mus musculus*	Comparative analysis of the kidney cell transcriptome in mice treated with low, intermediate and high doses of vancomycin.	[85]
Proteome	*Enterococcus sp.*	Proteomics analysis of environmental isolates of enterococcal species to search for biomarkers of vancomycin resistance in wild animal vectors.	[89]

I) Analysis of the Evolution of Vancomycin Resistance

The first study aimed at characterising the changes in gene expression associated with the evolution of resistance in pathogenic strains was reported in 2000, and involved a comparison of the total RNA isolated from the first clinical VRSA isolate Mu50 with a vancomycin susceptible strain Mu50Ω and a heterogenous intermediate resistance strain Mu3 [62]. Although the effectiveness of this early study was limited by the technology available for measuring the changes in gene expression (hybridisation to a plasmid library derived from shotgun cloning of genomic DNA and arrayed on a nylon membrane) it did provide the first evidence for the involvement of transcription of the response regulator *vraR* in modulating the level of vancomycin resistance in *S. aureus*, demonstrating a marked up-regulation of this gene in the two resistant strains. This was subsequently shown to be sufficient to increase the level of vancomycin resistance in a non-susceptible strain by engineering over-expression of *vraR* in *S. aureus* N315P. An association between up-regulation of expression of the *vraRS* two-component system and the evolution of vancomycin resistance in *S. aureus* was also uncovered in a transcriptome comparison involving strains from the Tomasz series of matched clinical isolates [39]. Using Affymetrix microarrays a total of 224 genes were identified as being significantly differently expressed between strain JH9 (vancomycin MIC = 8 µg/ml) and JH1 (vancomycin MIC = 1 µg/ml). Many of the genes identified have roles in cell envelope biogenesis, but a large proportion are housekeeping genes or genes with no known function and their significance in the evolution of resistance is still far from clear. This scenario has been repeated in many of the other studies from Table 3 i), with global observations highlighting changes in the expression of ca. 2-10% of the genome in each case but providing a rational hypothesis for only a minority of the genes identified, typically where they encode known cell wall associated functions [38, 63-69]. While this could be consistent with the changes in expression that are important for resistance taking place superimposed on a background of non-associated changes, it seems more likely that an incomplete understanding of the integration of gene expression with cellular metabolism means we are currently failing to properly recognise the significance of the observations being made. In addition, it is important to recognise that our knowledge of the mode of action of vancomycin may be incomplete. While it is highly specific for binding to the D-Ala-D-Ala termini of nascent peptidoglycan, a recent proteomics study using semi-synthetic photoaffinity labeled derivatives indicated secondary protein targets for vancomycin binding in both *S. aureus* and *E. faecalis* [70]. Interestingly, these included a peptide ABC transport protein in *E. faecalis* raising the possibility that vancomycin can impede the uptake of nutrients from the environment which could produce a knock-on effect on primary cellular metabolism. There is certainly also evidence for a complexity associated with the evolution of vancomycin resistance in *S. aureus* which has yet to be understood (see Howden *et al.* [71] for an extensive review). Comparison of the transcriptomes of multiple susceptible and non-susceptible clinical pairs of MRSA have indicated that the up-regulation of *vraS* and genes attributed to a cell wall stress stimulon is not essential for the acquisition of resistance [68], and analysis of the mutations arising during a laboratory evolution of resistance in a susceptible clinical isolate has also identified multiple routes to reduced vancomycin susceptibility [38]. Two strains generated by selection on agar plates containing vancomycin exhibited both different mutations from each other, and from the resistant isolate which ultimately developed in the clinical setting. Missense point mutations associated with the *walk* or *vraS* regulatory loci were present in the former, while the clinical isolate possessed a defect in *stp1* [38]. A final point to note when considering the results reported from different functional genomics studies is that interpretation can be hampered by significant differences in the way in which the experimental data have been collected. Gene expression is highly condition dependent and can vary both according to the growth media used, and with the cell density at which cultures are sampled. Vancomycin resistant isolates are sometimes grown for analysis in the presence of vancomycin, and sometimes in its absence, thus also introducing additional variables into the studies.

II) Construction and Analysis of Engineered Mutations to Define Their Roles in Resistance

Functional genomics analysis of the evolution of vancomycin resistance in bacterial strains isolated from patients in the clinic is clearly a challenging problem where the complex set of variables can confound a clear interpretation of the results. However, where it is possible to reduce the variables to a minimum, by for instance the genetic engineering of defined changes in gene expression, these types of studies can be interpreted with much greater confidence. The importance of candidate mutations identified in clinical studies have therefore often been tested in more detail by recreating the mutation in a clean genetic background and analysing the effects not only on phenotype but also on global gene expression (Table 3 ii)). In this way, the *vraSR* two-component regulatory system was shown to be required for the up-regulation of a subset of 46 genes whose transcription was induced following exposure of *S. aureus* N315 to vancomycin [72]. The role of the serine/threonine phosphatase *stp1* in vancomycin resistance in *S. aureus* has similarly been studied by construction and transcriptome analysis of a defined deletion mutant strain [36]. The effect on gene expression of an insertion mutation in *stp1* found in a clinical isolate has also been determined [38], but an integrated analysis of the two sets of results has not yet been reported. Howden *et al.* [33] conducted bi-directional allelic exchange experiments with the *walKR* regulatory locus in vancomycin susceptible and non-susceptible clinical MRSA isolates to verify linkage of missense point mutations in these genes with the resistance phenotype. Comparison of the transcriptomes of the engineered mutants with those of the parental strains identified 163 genes whose expression was reproducibly affected by the changes in *walKR*. Interestingly, these were dominated by functions associated with primary metabolism, while only a minority of genes from the *S. aureus* cell wall stimulon were identified. In *Listeria monocytogenes* and *Bacillus subtilis*, a comparison of the changes induced in the transcriptome or proteome following exposure to vancomycin in parent and deletion mutant strains has been used to define the role of alternative sigma factors in coordinating the response to the antibiotic treatment [73, 74].

III) Characterisation of the Changes in Gene Expression Induced by Vancomycin Treatment

The analysis of changes in the transcriptome or proteome has been used extensively in a wide variety of bacteria as a method for characterising their global responses to antibiotic stress. The goals of these types of studies have been two-fold: to characterise biomarkers or signature changes in expression that can serve as specific reporters for drug activity; and to define and understand the regulatory networks that orchestrate the cellular responses to antibiotic stress. Table 3 iii) lists those reports which have involved vancomycin. Considerable effort has been put into developing *B. subtilis* as a model system for Gram-positive bacteria (including staphylococci, streptococci and enterococci) to investigate the effect of known antibacterial compounds on bacterial gene expression [75-78]. The rationale behind this approach was to develop an extensive database of responses which can be used in comparisons to screen novel compounds both to assay for their efficacy as antibacterial agents, and to determine their specific mode of action. In this context the responses to vancomycin at the levels of transcription and protein synthesis have been recorded as expression signatures representative of the inhibition of cell wall biosynthesis. While this approach has yet to bear fruit in terms of drug discovery, it has provided a wealth of data useful for defining the regulatory networks important for coordinating adaptation to antibiotic insult in *B. subtilis*. Similar experiments have been performed (but to a more limited extent) to address specific questions concerning drug activity in other bacterial strains [79-84]. To understand the mechanisms used to maintain cell envelope homeostasis in *Mycobacterium tuberculosis* and thereby identify potential targets for new anti-TB drugs, Proveddi *et al.* characterised the variation in the transcriptional response to inhibitory and subinhibitory concentrations of vancomycin [84]. The results reinforced the importance of the alternative sigma factor σE for conferring a basal level resistance to vancomycin, and identified a small number of candidate genes for further study. The σE regulon was also found to play a central role in coordinating the response to the inhibition of cell wall biosynthesis in *S. coelicolor*, along with elements of the stringent response and the osmotic and oxidative stress regulons [82]. By characterising the transcriptional responses to vancomycin, bacitracin and moenomycin which each inhibit different targets in peptidoglycan biosynthesis it was possible for the authors to identify both common and compound-specific responses. *S. coelicolor* possesses inducible VanB-type resistance to vancomycin but the results highlighted changes in expression of ca. 25% of the genome following exposure to the antibiotic and indicated the importance of generalised stress response systems which may serve to enable the cells to survive until the specific resistance mechanisms become fully functional. Comparative transcriptome studies have also been undertaken in *S. aureus* to more specifically characterise the modes of action of two antibiotics that are active against vancomycin resistant MRSA strains [81, 83]. In one study, the global response of *S. aureus* to telavancin, a semisynthetic lipoglycopeptide derivative of vancomycin, was compared with the changes induced by the parent compound vancomycin, a lipid II inhibitor enduracidin, and a membrane depolarising agent carbonyl cyanide m-chlorophenylhydrazone (CCCP) [83]. The results indicated that telavancin not only causes a strong inhibition of peptidoglycan biosynthesis comparable to vancomycin, but also produces a sustained membrane depolarisation effect. This dual activity offers an explanation for its increased potency. Muthailyan *et al.* [81] similarly compared the response of *S. aureus* to the lipopeptide antibiotic daptomycin with those induced by vancomycin, CCCP and nisin to more fully characterise its mode of action. Daptomycin exhibits activity against vancomycin-resistant strains, and the observation that it induces the expression of genes characteristic of both the response to membrane depolarisation and to the inhibition of peptidoglycan biosynthesis again suggests a more complex mode of action than for vancomycin.

IV) Miscellaneous Studies on Other Aspects of Vancomycin Resistance and Activity

The use of vancomycin in the clinic has been purposely restricted over the years not only to minimise the occurrence of resistance and prolong its useful therapeutic lifespan, but also because it is nephrotoxic. A functional genomics approach has been used in a study designed to gain insight into the molecular basis of this nephrotoxicity, and to evaluate gene biomarkers of vancomycin-induced kidney damage [85]. Using the mouse as a model system, vancomycin was administered in a range of doses by both intravenous (IV) and intraperitoneal (IP) routes and the effect on the kidney transcriptome analysed after eight days of treatment. The analysis identified a greater response to the antibiotic following IP administration, and provided evidence to support the use of certain gene markers of kidney toxicity. Furthermore, analysis of the common response to the highest dose of vancomycin (400 mg/kg) independent of the method of administration was suggestive of oxidative stress and mitochondrial damage in vancomycin induced toxicity. The mouse has also been used as a model to investigate the effect that vancomycin may have on the gut microbiota, and the relationship of this with host metabolism [86]. In the only metabolomics study that could be found in this review of the literature, changes in the metabolites present in faecal and urine samples taken from mice treated with vancomycin were analysed as markers of host metabolism, and compared to changes in gut microbiota as determined by analysis of 16S rRNA sequences. Clear differences in gut microbial communities between control and vancomycin treated mice were observed, together with concomitant changes in the excretion of metabolites from the host including uracil, amino acids and short chain fatty acids.

The success of *E. faecalis* in nosocomial infections is in part attributable to its ability to grow and colonise many hostile environments including the gastrointestinal tract. Bile acids are a major stress factor in this environment, and the response of the vancomycin resistant *E. faecalis* strain V583 to the presence of bile acids has been analysed by measuring changes in the proteome and transcriptome [87, 88]. The data provided an overview of the processes that *E. faecalis* must regulate in order to survive and adapt to a bile-rich environment, and these included fatty acid and phopsholipid pathways which were significantly down-regulated in response to bile.

While vancomycin use in the clinic has been carefully controlled, it has seen extensive use in the past for agricultural purposes. This has resulted in a widespread exposure to vancomycin in the environment, raising the likelihood of the formation of reservoirs of bacterial resistance hosted in wild animal populations. Proteomics approaches are being used to begin to investigate and address this problem, analysing the proteomes of vancomycin resistant enterococcal strains isolated from seagull faecal samples to search for biomarkers with the potential to conveniently track the occurrence and spread of the resistant strains [89, 90].

Conclusion

Comparative and functional genomics are still relatively recent approaches for scientific investigation, and there is undoubtedly room for improving their effectiveness as tools for solving complex biological questions. Nevertheless it is clear that their use, backed up by more focused biochemical and molecular genetic studies, is already yielding important new insights into both the activity of vancomycin, and the evolution of bacterial resistance towards it. The dramatic impacts on pathogen physiology of the relatively few mutations that arise during treatment of some persistent MRSA infections with vancomycin has in particular become evident, although the underlying mechanisms are yet to be fully established. The incidence of vancomycin resistant pathogens in hospital acquired infections is on an upward trend and there is a continued need for understanding the mechanisms, origin, evolution and transmission of resistance. The current inadequacies in the development and supply of new antibacterial treatments for the clinic further emphasises the need to understand the resistance developing towards the antibiotics already in use. Such knowledge could not only help to prolong the useful lifespan of an antibiotic, but may also suggest ways in which the next generation of antibacterial compounds can be designed or improved. To better achieve this goal it will be important to look more holistically at the evolution of resistance than has thus far been attempted. The evident complexities of intermediate level vancomycin resistance in MRSA strains point towards a need for a more complete understanding of the relationship between genotype and phenotype that will require an integrated network analysis of data collected on all –omic levels from genome through to metabolome via the interactome. Analysis of the metabolome in resistant strains has notably been lacking in the studies reported to date, despite the number of reports highlighting major changes in the expression of genes encoding functions associated with primary metabolism during the development of resistance. Current evidence that acquisition of intermediate resistance in MRSA can involve several independent mutagenic routes – via *vraSR*, *graSR*, *walKR* or *stil* – would be put into a more usefully interpretable context if the corresponding changes in the metabolome were known. Indeed, a systems biology strategy in which quantitative –omics measurements are viewed and interpreted in the context of a detailed knowledge of the cellular protein-DNA and protein-protein interaction networks would offer a powerful approach for understanding how resistance to vancomycin arises. There is also much that could usefully be learned through a similarly more integrated analysis of the other aspects of vancomycin activity which have been the subject of the studies reviewed in this chapter. The basis of the toxicity of vancomycin in humans remains poorly defined, as do the factors important for resistant strains to succeed in their host environments. Characterisation of the responses to vancomycin in non-pathogenic Gram-positive model organisms also offers the opportunity to more safely explore fundamental aspects of the mechanisms important for resistance, and to search for biomarkers or reporters which may be useful in discovering future antibacterial activities. Analysis of the vancomycin inducible resistance system in *S. coelicolor* in particular has yielded useful mechanistic insights [58, 60, 61, 91, 92].

Comparative and functional genomics analysis has had less of an impact on the understanding of vancomycin resistance in enterococci, where the evolution of resistance is usually associated with the acquisition of one of only a few well characterised resistance gene functions via horizontal gene transfer. Interestingly however, the focus in the enterococcal studies has been more on the assessment of the types of resistant strains present in community and hospital settings, and in the wider natural environment. Investigations into the genomic factors which may promote the transfer and acquisition of resistance genes, or potentiate their expression once acquired, are starting to be complemented by surveys of strains prevalent in healthy and diseased individuals, and in reservoir vector species such as wild birds. Further similar efforts will be required to more fully understand the evolution of predominant clones and species in the different hosts and environments, particularly the hospital environment. Evidence supporting the transfer of *vanA* resistance genes from enterococci to *S. aureus* strains to produce fully vancomycin resistant VRSA [93, 94] makes this task even more important. In this context the development of methodologies to enable studies of mixed microbial species in wound or wound model settings could more realistically reflect the evolution of vancomycin resistance in the clinic. Significant technical challenges have imposed important limitations on the studies reviewed in this chapter, but advances currently being made are promising ways in which these will be overcome to open up new, more insightful possibilities for the future. The ability to reliably make single cell —omics measurements [95, 96] should eventually replace the existing requirement to sample large unsynchronized populations of cells grown under artificial laboratory conditions. The ability to analyse a single cell obtained from any environment would greatly improve the sensitivity and confidence with which quantitative measurements of gene expression or metabolite concentration (which are averaged out in samples from populations) can be linked to differences in gene sequence or content.

Much will depend on the success of technological advances being made in quantitative biology, and on improving computational techniques for integrating and interpreting large–omics datasets, but the tools to provide the knowledgebase for helping push back the tide of bacterial resistance to antibiotics could be on the horizon. Furthermore, the ability to rapidly sequence strains causing an antibiotic resistant infection, coupled with a detailed understanding of the genotype-phenotype relationship, may in future offer the opportunity for treatment regimes to be tailored to the needs of individual cases.

References

[1] Levy, S.; Marshall, B. Antibacterial resistance worldwide: causes, challenges and responses. *Nature medicine*. 2004; 10(12 Suppl):9.

[2] Davies, J.; Davies, D. Origins and evolution of antibiotic resistance. *Microbiology and molecular biology reviews : MMBR*. 2010; 74(3):417-33.

[3] Levine, D. P. Vancomycin: A History. *Clinical Infectious Diseases*. 2006; 42(Supplementary):S5-12.

[4] Barna, J. C.; Williams DH. The structure and mode of action of glycopeptide antibiotics of the vancomycin group. *Annu. Rev. Microbiol.* 1984; 38:339-57.

[5] Spellberg, B.; Guidos, R.; Gilbert, D.; Bradley, J.; Boucher, H. W.; Scheld, W. M. et al. The epidemic of antibiotic-resistant infections: a call to action for the medical community from the Infectious Diseases Society of America. *Clin. Infect. Dis.* 2008; 46(2):155-64.

[6] Howden, B.; Davies, J.; Johnson, P.; Stinear, T.; Grayson, M. Reduced vancomycin susceptibility in *Staphylococcus aureus*, including vancomycin-intermediate and heterogeneous vancomycin-intermediate strains: resistance mechanisms, laboratory detection, and clinical implications. *Clinical microbiology reviews*. 2010; 23(1):99-139.

[7] Lagesen, K.; Ussery, D.; Wassenaar, T. Genome update: the 1000th genome--a cautionary tale. *Microbiology (Reading, England)*. 2010; 156(Pt 3):603-8.

[8] Meyerson, M.; Gabriel, S.; Getz, G. Advances in understanding cancer genomes through second-generation sequencing. *Nat. Rev. Genet.* 2010; 11(10):685-96.

[9]   Cooper, G. M.; Shendure, J. Needles in stacks of needles: finding disease-causal variants in a wealth of genomic data. *Nat. Rev. Genet.* 2011; 12(9):628-40.

[10] Morrell, P.; Buckler, E.; Ross-Ibarra, J. Crop genomics: advances and applications. *Nature reviews Genetics.* 2011; 13(2):85-96.

[11] Groenen, M. A.; Archibald, A. L.; Uenishi, H.; Tuggle, C. K.; Takeuchi, Y.; Rothschild, M. F. et al. Analyses of pig genomes provide insight into porcine demography and evolution. *Nature.* 2012; 491(7424):393-8.

[12] Dekkers, J. C. Application of genomics tools to animal breeding. *Curr. Genomics.* 2012; 13(3):207-12.

[13] Binnewies, T.; Motro, Y; Hallin, P.; Lund, O.; Dunn, D.; La, T. et al. Ten years of bacterial genome sequencing: comparative-genomics-based discoveries. *Functional & integrative genomics.* 2006; 6(3):165-85.

[14] Harris, S.; Cartwright, E.; Torok, M.; Holden, M.; Brown, N.; Ogilvy-Stuart, A. et al. Whole-genome sequencing for analysis of an outbreak of meticillin-resistant *Staphylococcus aureus*: a descriptive study. *The Lancet infectious diseases.* 2013; 13(2):130-6.

[15] Hung, W. C.; Takano, T.; Higuchi, W.; Iwao, Y.; Khokhlova, O.; Teng, L. J. et al. Comparative genomics of community-acquired ST59 methicillin-resistant *Staphylococcus aureus* in Taiwan: novel mobile resistance structures with IS1216V. *PLoS One.* 2012; 7(10):e46987.

[16] Yamamoto, T.; Takano, T.; Higuchi, W.; Iwao, Y.; Singur, O.; Reva, I. et al. Comparative genomics and drug resistance of a geographic variant of ST239 methicillin-resistant *Staphylococcus aureus* emerged in Russia. *PLoS One.* 2012; 7(1):e29187.

[17] Feng, Y.; Chen, C. J.; Su, L. H.; Hu, S.; Yu, J.; Chiu, C. H. Evolution and pathogenesis of *Staphylococcus aureus*: lessons learned from genotyping and comparative genomics. *FEMS Microbiol. Rev.* 2008; 32(1):23-37.

[18] Iwao, Y.; Ishii, R.; Tomita, Y.; Shibuya, Y.; Takano, T.; Hung, W. C. et al. The emerging ST8 methicillin-resistant *Staphylococcus aureus* clone in the community in Japan: associated infections, genetic diversity, and comparative genomics. *J. Infect. Chemother.* 2012; 18(2):228-40.

[19] Kuroda, M.; Ohta, T.; Uchiyama, I.; Baba, T.; Yuzawa, H.; Kobayashi, I. et al. Whole genome sequencing of meticillin-resistant *Staphylococcus aureus. Lancet.* 2001; 357(9264):1225-40.

[20] Hiramatsu, K.; Hanaki, H.; Ino, T.; Yabuta, K.; Oguri, T.; Tenover, F. Methicillin-resistant *Staphylococcus aureus* clinical strain with reduced

vancomycin susceptibility. *The Journal of antimicrobial chemotherapy.* 1997; 40(1):135-6.

[21] Kuwahara-Arai, K.; Kondo, N.; Hori, S. Tateda-Suzuki E, Hiramatsu K. Suppression of methicillin resistance in a mecA-containing pre-methicillin-resistant *Staphylococcus aureus* strain is caused by the mecI-mediated repression of PBP 2' production. *Antimicrobial agents and chemotherapy.* 1996; 40(12):2680-5.

[22] Hanaki, H.; Kuwahara-Arai, K.; Boyle-Vavra, S.; Daum, R. S.; Labischinski, H.; Hiramatsu, K. Activated cell-wall synthesis is associated with vancomycin resistance in methicillin-resistant *Staphylococcus aureus* clinical strains Mu3 and Mu50. *J. Antimicrob. Chemother.* 1998; 42(2):199-209.

[23] Hanaki, H.; Labischinski, H.; Inaba, Y.; Kondo, N.; Murakami, H.; Hiramatsu, K. Increase in glutamine-non-amidated muropeptides in the peptidoglycan of vancomycin-resistant *Staphylococcus aureus* strain Mu50. *J. Antimicrob. Chemother.* 1998; 42(3):315-20.

[24] Cui, L.; Murakami, H.; Kuwahara-Arai, K.; Hanaki, H.; Hiramatsu, K. Contribution of a thickened cell wall and its glutamine nonamidated component to the vancomycin resistance expressed by *Staphylococcus aureus* Mu50. *Antimicrob. Agents Chemother.* 2000; 44(9):2276-85.

[25] Avison, M.; Bennett, P.; Howe, R.; Walsh, T. Preliminary analysis of the genetic basis for vancomycin resistance in *Staphylococcus aureus* strain Mu50. *The Journal of antimicrobial chemotherapy.* 2002; 49(2):255-60.

[26] Ohta, T.; Hirakawa, H.; Morikawa, K.; Maruyama, A.; Inose, Y.; Yamashita, A. et al. Nucleotide substitutions in *Staphylococcus aureus* strains, Mu50, Mu3, and N315. *DNA research : an international journal for rapid publication of reports on genes and genomes.* 2004; 11(1):51-6.

[27] Belcheva, A.; Verma, V.; Golemi-Kotra, D. DNA-binding activity of the vancomycin resistance associated regulator protein VraR and the role of phosphorylation in transcriptional regulation of the *vraSR* operon. *Biochemistry.* 2009; 48(24):5592-601.

[28] Belcheva, A.; Golemi-Kotra, D. A close-up view of the VraSR two-component system. A mediator of *Staphylococcus aureus* response to cell wall damage. *The Journal of biological chemistry.* 2008; 283(18):12354-64.

[29] Belcheva, A.; Verma, V.; Korenevsky, A.; Fridman, M.; Kumar, K.; Golemi-Kotra, D. Roles of DNA sequence and sigma A factor in

transcription of the *vraSR* operon. *Journal of bacteriology*. 2012; 194(1):61-71.

[30] Pane-Farre, J.; Jonas, B.; Forstner, K.; Engelmann, S.; Hecker, M. The sigmaB regulon in *Staphylococcus aureus* and its regulation. *Int. J. Med. Microbiol.* 2006; 296(4-5):237-58.

[31] Mwangi, M.; Wu, S.; Zhou, Y.; Sieradzki, K.; de Lencastre, H.; Richardson, P. et al. Tracking the *in vivo* evolution of multidrug resistance in *Staphylococcus aureus* by whole-genome sequencing. *Proceedings of the National Academy of Sciences of the United States of America.* 2007; 104(22):9451-6.

[32] Howden, B.; Stinear, T.; Allen, D.; Johnson, P.; Ward, P.; Davies, J. Genomic analysis reveals a point mutation in the two-component sensor gene *graS* that leads to intermediate vancomycin resistance in clinical *Staphylococcus aureus*. *Antimicrobial agents and chemotherapy.* 2008; 52(10):3755-62.

[33] Howden, B.; McEvoy, C.; Allen, D.; Chua, K.; Gao, W.; Harrison, P. et al. Evolution of multidrug resistance during *Staphylococcus aureus* infection involves mutation of the essential two component regulator WalKR. *PLoS pathogens.* 2011; 7(11).

[34] Cui, L.; Neoh, H-m.; Shoji, M.; Hiramatsu, K. Contribution of *vraSR* and *graSR* point mutations to vancomycin resistance in vancomycin-intermediate *Staphylococcus aureus*. *Antimicrobial agents and chemotherapy.* 2009; 53(3):1231-4.

[35] Neoh, H-m.; Cui, L.; Yuzawa, H.; Takeuchi, F.; Matsuo, M.; Hiramatsu, K. Mutated response regulator *graR* is responsible for phenotypic conversion of *Staphylococcus aureus* from heterogeneous vancomycin-intermediate resistance to vancomycin-intermediate resistance. *Antimicrobial agents and chemotherapy.* 2008; 52(1):45-53.

[36] Cameron, D.; Ward, D.; Kostoulias, X.; Howden, B.; Moellering, R.; Eliopoulos, G. et al. Serine/threonine phosphatase Stp1 contributes to reduced susceptibility to vancomycin and virulence in *Staphylococcus aureus*. *The Journal of infectious diseases.* 2012; 205(11):1677-87.

[37] Kos, V.; Desjardins, C.; Griggs, A.; Cerqueira, G.; Van Tonder, A.; Holden, M. et al. Comparative genomics of vancomycin-resistant *Staphylococcus aureus* strains and their positions within the clade most commonly associated with Methicillin-resistant *S. aureus* hospital-acquired infection in the United States. *mBio.* 2012; 3(3).

[38] Passalacqua, K.; Satola, S.; Crispell, E.; Read, T. A mutation in the PP2C phosphatase gene in a Staphylococcus aureus USA300 clinical

isolate with reduced susceptibility to vancomycin and daptomycin. *Antimicrobial agents and chemotherapy.* 2012; 56(10):5212-23.

[39] McAleese, F.; Wu, S.; Sieradzki, K.; Dunman, P.; Murphy, E.; Projan, S. et al. Overexpression of genes of the cell wall stimulon in clinical isolates of *Staphylococcus aureus* exhibiting vancomycin-intermediate-*S. aureus*-type resistance to vancomycin. *Journal of bacteriology.* 2006; 188(3):1120-33.

[40] Mwangi, M. M.; Wu, S. W.; Zhou, Y.; Sieradzki, K.; de Lencastre, H.; Richardson, P. et al. Tracking the in vivo evolution of multidrug resistance in *Staphylococcus aureus* by whole-genome sequencing. *Proc. Natl. Acad. Sci. U S A.* 2007; 104(22):9451-6.

[41] Sieradzki, K.; Leski, T.; Dick, J.; Borio, L.; Tomasz, A. Evolution of a vancomycin-intermediate *Staphylococcus aureus* strain in vivo: multiple changes in the antibiotic resistance phenotypes of a single lineage of methicillin-resistant *S. aureus* under the impact of antibiotics administered for chemotherapy. *J. Clin. Microbiol.* 2003; 41(4):1687-93.

[42] Klevens, R. M.; Morrison, M. A.; Nadle, J.; Petit, S.; Gershman, K.; Ray, S. et al. Invasive methicillin-resistant *Staphylococcus aureus* infections in the United States. *JAMA.* 2007; 298(15):1763-71.

[43] Werner, G.; Coque, T. M.; Franz, C. M.; Grohmann, E.; Hegstad, K.; Jensen, L. et al. Antibiotic resistant enterococci-Tales of a drug resistance gene trafficker. *Int. J. Med. Microbiol.* 2013.

[44] Palmer, K.; Kos, V.; Gilmore, M. Horizontal gene transfer and the genomics of enterococcal antibiotic resistance. *Current opinion in microbiology.* 2010; 13(5):632-9.

[45] Arias, C. A.; Murray, B. E. The rise of the Enterococcus: beyond vancomycin resistance. *Nat. Rev. Microbiol.* 2012; 10(4):266-78.

[46] Paulsen, I. T.; Banerjei, L.; Myers, G. S.; Nelson, K. E.; Seshadri, R.; Read, T. D. et al. Role of mobile DNA in the evolution of vancomycin-resistant *Enterococcus faecalis. Science.* 2003; 299(5615):2071-4.

[47] Shankar, N.; Baghdayan, A. S.; Gilmore, M. S. Modulation of virulence within a pathogenicity island in vancomycin-resistant *Enterococcus faecalis. Nature.* 2002; 417(6890):746-50.

[48] Lam, M.; Seemann, T.; Bulach, D.; Gladman, S.; Chen, H,.; Haring, V. et al. Comparative analysis of the first complete *Enterococcus faecium* genome. *Journal of bacteriology.* 2012; 194(9):2334-41.

[49] Palmer, K. L.; Carniol, K.; Manson, J. M.; Heiman, D.; Shea, T.; Young, S. et al. High-quality draft genome sequences of 28 Enterococcus sp. isolates. *J. Bacteriol.* 2010; 192(9):2469-70.

[50] Qin, X.; Galloway-Pena, J.; Sillanpaa, J.; Roh, J.; Nallapareddy, S.; Chowdhury, S. et al. Complete genome sequence of *Enterococcus faecium* strain TX16 and comparative genomic analysis of *Enterococcus faecium* genomes. *BMC microbiology.* 2012; 12:135.

[51] van Schaik, W.; Top, J.; Riley, D.; Boekhorst, J.; Vrijenhoek, J.; Schapendonk, C. et al. Pyrosequencing-based comparative genome analysis of the nosocomial pathogen *Enterococcus faecium* and identification of a large transferable pathogenicity island. *BMC Genomics.* 2010; 11:239.

[52] Johnson, P.; Ballard, S.; Grabsch, E.; Stinear, T.; Seemann, T.; Young, H. et al. A sustained hospital outbreak of vancomycin-resistant *Enterococcus faecium* bacteremia due to emergence of *vanB E. faecium* sequence type 203. *The Journal of infectious diseases.* 2010; 202(8): 1278-86.

[53] Solheim, M.; Brekke, M. C.; Snipen, L. G.; Willems, R. J.; Nes, I. F.; Brede, D. A. Comparative genomic analysis reveals significant enrichment of mobile genetic elements and genes encoding surface structure-proteins in hospital-associated clonal complex 2 *Enterococcus faecalis. BMC Microbiol.* 2011; 11:3.

[54] Palmer, K. L.; Godfrey, P.; Griggs, A.; Kos, V. N.; Zucker, J.; Desjardins, C. et al. Comparative genomics of enterococci: variation in *Enterococcus faecalis*, clade structure in *E. faecium*, and defining characteristics of *E. gallinarum* and *E. casseliflavus. mBio.* 2012; 3(1):e00318-11.

[55] Palmer, K. L.; Gilmore, M. S. Multidrug-resistant enterococci lack CRISPR-cas. *mBio.* 2010; 1(4).

[56] Santagati, M.; Campanile, F.; Stefani, S. Genomic diversification of enterococci in hosts: the role of the mobilome. *Front Microbiol.* 2012; 3:95.

[57] Guardabassi, L,; Perichon, B.; van Heijenoort, J.; Blanot, D.; Courvalin, P. Glycopeptide resistance *vanA* operons in *Paenibacillus* strains isolated from soil. *Antimicrob. Agents Chemother.* 2005; 49(10): 4227-33.

[58] Koteva, K.; Hong, H. J.; Wang, X. D.; Nazi, I.; Hughes, D.; Naldrett, M. J. et al. A vancomycin photoprobe identifies the histidine kinase VanSsc as a vancomycin receptor. *Nat. Chem. Biol.* 2010; 6(5):327-9.

[59] Hong, H-J. Studying gene induction of glycopeptide resistance using gene swapping. *Methods in molecular biology (Clifton, NJ).* 2010; 642:45-62.

[60] Hutchings, M. I.; Hong, H. J.; Buttner, M. J. The vancomycin resistance VanRS two-component signal transduction system of *Streptomyces coelicolor*. *Mol. Microbiol*. 2006; 59(3):923-35.

[61] Novotna, G.; Hill, C.; Vincent, K.; Liu, C.; Hong, H. J. A novel membrane protein, VanJ, conferring resistance to teicoplanin. *Antimicrob. Agents Chemother*. 2012; 56(4):1784-96.

[62] Kuroda, M.; Kuwahara-Arai, K.; Hiramatsu, K. Identification of the up- and down-regulated genes in vancomycin-resistant *Staphylococcus aureus* strains Mu3 and Mu50 by cDNA differential hybridization method. *Biochem. Biophys. Res. Commun*. 2000; 269(2):485-90.

[63] Scherl, A.; Francois, P.; Charbonnier, Y.; Deshusses, J.; Koessler, T.; Huyghe, A. et al. Exploring glycopeptide-resistance in *Staphylococcus aureus*: a combined proteomics and transcriptomics approach for the identification of resistance-related markers. *BMC Genomics*. 2006; 7:296.

[64] Haas, W.; Kaushal, D.; Sublett, J.; Obert, C.; Tuomanen, E. Vancomycin stress response in a sensitive and a tolerant strain of *Streptococcus pneumoniae*. *Journal of bacteriology*. 2005; 187(23):8205-10.

[65] Pieper, R.; Gatlin-Bunai, C.; Mongodin, E.; Parmar, P.; Huang, S-T.; Clark, D. et al. Comparative proteomic analysis of *Staphylococcus aureus* strains with differences in resistance to the cell wall-targeting antibiotic vancomycin. *Proteomics*. 2006; 6(15):4246-58.

[66] Gatlin, C.; Pieper, R.; Huang, S-T.; Mongodin, E.; Gebregeorgis, E.; Parmar, P. et al. Proteomic profiling of cell envelope-associated proteins from *Staphylococcus aureus*. *Proteomics*. 2006; 6(5):1530-49.

[67] Drummelsmith, J.; Winstall, E.; Bergeron, M.; Poirier, G.; Ouellette, M. Comparative proteomics analyses reveal a potential biomarker for the detection of vancomycin-intermediate *Staphylococcus aureus* strains. *Journal of proteome research*. 2007; 6(12):4690-702.

[68] Howden, B.; Smith, D.; Mansell, A.; Johnson, P.; Ward, P.; Stinear, T. et al. Different bacterial gene expression patterns and attenuated host immune responses are associated with the evolution of low-level vancomycin resistance during persistent methicillin-resistant *Staphylococcus aureus* bacteraemia. *BMC microbiology*. 2008; 8:39.

[69] Wang, X.; He, X.; Jiang, Z.; Wang, J.; Chen, X.; Liu, D. et al. Proteomic analysis of the *Enterococcus faecalis* V583 strain and clinical isolate V309 under vancomycin treatment. *Journal of proteome research*. 2010; 9(4):1772-85.

[70] Eirich, Jr.; Orth, R.; Sieber, S. Unraveling the protein targets of vancomycin in living *S. aureus* and *E. faecalis* cells. *Journal of the American Chemical Society.* 2011; 133(31):12144-53.

[71] Howden, B.; Peleg, A.; Stinear, T. The Evolution of Vancomycin Intermediate *Staphylococcus aureus* (VISA) and Heterogenous-VISA. *Infection, genetics and evolution : Journal of molecular epidemiology and evolutionary genetics in infectious diseases.* 2013.

[72] Kuroda, M.; Kuroda, H.; Oshima, T.; Takeuchi, F.; Mori, H.; Hiramatsu, K. Two-component system VraSR positively modulates the regulation of cell-wall biosynthesis pathway in *Staphylococcus aureus*. *Molecular microbiology.* 2003; 49(3):807-21.

[73] Shin, J-H.; Kim, J.; Kim, S-M.; Kim, S.; Lee, J-C.; Ahn, J-M. et al. sigmaB-dependent protein induction in *Listeria monocytogenes* during vancomycin stress. *FEMS Microbiology Letters.* 2010; 308(1):94-100.

[74] Eiamphungporn, W.; Helmann, J. The *Bacillus subtilis* sigma(M) regulon and its contribution to cell envelope stress responses. *Molecular microbiology.* 2008; 67(4):830-48.

[75] Bandow, J.; Brotz, H.; Leichert, L.; Labischinski, H.; Hecker, M. Proteomic approach to understanding antibiotic action. *Antimicrobial agents and chemotherapy.* 2003; 47(3):948-55.

[76] Cao, M.; Wang, T.; Ye, R.; Helmann, J. Antibiotics that inhibit cell wall biosynthesis induce expression of the *Bacillus subtilis* sigma(W) and sigma(M) regulons. *Molecular microbiology.* 2002; 45(5):1267-76.

[77] Hutter, B.; Schaab, C.; Albrecht, S.; Borgmann, M.; Brunner, N.; Freiberg, C. et al. Prediction of mechanisms of action of antibacterial compounds by gene expression profiling. *Antimicrobial agents and chemotherapy.* 2004; 48(8):2838-44.

[78] Freiberg, C.; Fischer, H.; Brunner, N. Discovering the mechanism of action of novel antibacterial agents through transcriptional profiling of conditional mutants. *Antimicrobial agents and chemotherapy.* 2005; 49(2):749-59.

[79] McCallum, N.; Spehar, G.; Bischoff, M.; Berger-Bachi, B. Strain dependence of the cell wall-damage induced stimulon in *Staphylococcus aureus. Biochimica et biophysica acta.* 2006; 1760(10):1475-81.

[80] Wecke, T.; Veith, B.; Ehrenreich, A.; Mascher, T. Cell envelope stress response in *Bacillus licheniformis*: integrating comparative genomics, transcriptional profiling, and regulon mining to decipher a complex regulatory network. *Journal of bacteriology.* 2006; 188(21):7500-11.

[81] Muthaiyan, A.; Silverman, J.; Jayaswal, R.; Wilkinson, B. Transcriptional profiling reveals that daptomycin induces the *Staphylococcus aureus* cell wall stress stimulon and genes responsive to membrane depolarization. *Antimicrobial agents and chemotherapy.* 2008; 52(3):980-90.

[82] Hesketh, A.; Hill, C.; Mokhtar, J.; Novotna, G.; Tran, N.; Bibb, M. et al. Genome-wide dynamics of a bacterial response to antibiotics that target the cell envelope. *BMC Genomics.* 2011; 12:226.

[83] Song, Y.; Lunde, C.; Benton, B.; Wilkinson, B. Further insights into the mode of action of the lipoglycopeptide telavancin through global gene expression studies. *Antimicrobial agents and chemotherapy.* 2012; 56(6):3157-64.

[84] Provvedi, R.; Boldrin, F.; Falciani, F.; Palu, G.; Manganelli, R. Global transcriptional response to vancomycin in *Mycobacterium tuberculosis*. *Microbiology (Reading, England).* 2009; 155(Pt 4):1093-102.

[85] Dieterich, C.; Puey, A.; Lin, S.; Lyn, S.; Swezey, R.; Furimsky, A. et al. Gene expression analysis reveals new possible mechanisms of vancomycin-induced nephrotoxicity and identifies gene markers candidates. *Toxicological sciences : an official journal of the Society of Toxicology.* 2009; 107(1):258-69.

[86] Yap, I.; Li, J.; Saric, J.; Martin, F-P.; Davies, H.; Wang, Y. et al. Metabonomic and microbiological analysis of the dynamic effect of vancomycin-induced gut microbiota modification in the mouse. *Journal of proteome research.* 2008; 7(9):3718-28.

[87] Solheim, M.; Aakra, A.; Vebo, H.; Snipen, L.; Nes, I. Transcriptional responses of *Enterococcus faecalis* V583 to bovine bile and sodium dodecyl sulfate. *Applied and environmental microbiology.* 2007; 73(18):5767-74.

[88] Bohle, L.; Faergestad, E.; Veiseth-Kent, E.; Steinmoen, H.; Nes, I.; Eijsink, V. et al. Identification of proteins related to the stress response in *Enterococcus faecalis* V583 caused by bovine bile. *Proteome science.* 2010; 8:37.

[89] Radhouani, H.; Poeta, P.; Pinto, L.; Monteiro, R.; Nunes-Miranda, J.; Correia, S. et al. Comparative proteomic map among *vanA*-containing Enterococcus isolated from yellow-legged gulls. *Journal of Integrated OMICS.* 2012; 2.

[90] Radhouani, H.; Poeta, P.; Pinto, L.; Miranda, J. l.; Coelho, C. l.; Carvalho, C. et al. Proteomic characterization of *vanA*-containing

Enterococcus recovered from Seagulls at the Berlengas Natural Reserve, W Portugal. *Proteome science.* 2010; 8:48.

[91] Hong, H. J.; Hutchings, M. I.; Hill. L. M.; Buttner, M. J. The role of the novel Fem protein VanK in vancomycin resistance in *Streptomyces coelicolor. J. Biol. Chem.* 2005; 280(13):13055-61.

[92] Hong, H. J.; Hutchings, M. I.; Neu, J. M.; Wright, G. D.; Paget, M. S.; Buttner, M. J. Characterization of an inducible vancomycin resistance system in *Streptomyces coelicolor* reveals a novel gene (*vanK*) required for drug resistance. *Mol. Microbiol.* 2004; 52(4):1107-21.

[93] Leclercq, R.; Derlot, E.; Duval, J.; Courvalin, P. Plasmid-mediated resistance to vancomycin and teicoplanin in *Enterococcus faecium. N. Engl. J. Med.* 1988; 319(3):157-61.

[94] Uttley, A. H.; Collins, C. H.; Naidoo, J.; George, R. C. Vancomycin-resistant enterococci. *Lancet.* 1988; 1(8575-6):57-8.

[95] Wang, D.; Bodovitz, S. Single cell analysis: the new frontier in 'omics'. *Trends Biotechnol.* 2010; 28(6):281-90.

[96] Fritzsch, F. S.; Dusny, C.; Frick, O.; Schmid, A. Single-cell analysis in biotechnology, systems biology, and biocatalysis. *Annu. Rev. Chem. Biomol. Eng.* 2012; 3:129-55.

In: Vancomycin   ISBN: 978-1-62948-559-1
Editor: Abu Gafar Hossion   © 2013 Nova Science Publishers, Inc.

Chapter 3

Vancomycin: Use, Dosing and Therapeutic Drug Monitoring

*Iris Usach, Virginia Melis and Jose-Esteban Peris**
Department of Pharmacy and Pharmaceutical Technology,
Faculty of Pharmacy, University of Valencia, Valencia, Spain

Abstract

Vancomycin is frequently used for the treatment of serious gram-positive infections involving methicillin-resistant *Staphylococcus aureus* (MRSA). It is also used for the treatment of infections caused by gram-positive microorganisms in patients with serious allergies to beta-lactam antibiotics and for the treatment of pseudomembranous colitis caused by the bacterium *Clostridium difficile*. Although early use of vancomycin was associated with nephrotoxicity and ototoxicity, it appears that impurities in early formulations were responsible, at least in part, for these toxic effects. To treat systemic infections, vancomycin must be administered intravenously. The intramuscular route is not used due to possible tissue necrosis. Vancomycin is not absorbed when it is orally administered, and this administration route is only used for the treatment of pseudomembranous colitis. The serum vancomycin concentration-time profile is complex and has been described with one-, two-, and three-compartment pharmacokinetic models. In patients with normal renal

* Corresponding author: jose.e.peris@uv.es.

function, the terminal half-life ranges from 6 to 12 hours and the volume of distribution ranges from 0.4 to 1 L/kg. Several studies have indicated that vancomycin is a time-dependent (concentration-independent) killer of gram-positive pathogens, and that the best determinant of efficacy is the ratio of the area under the serum drug concentration-versus-time curve and the minimum inhibitory concentration (AUC/MIC). An AUC/MIC ratio equal to or above 400 has been recommended as target to achieve clinical effectiveness. Different vancomycin initial dosing schedules have been recommended for adults with impaired renal function, pediatric patients and neonates. Subsequent dosing should be adjusted based on serum vancomycin levels, using the AUC/MIC ratio as target, or trough concentrations as a surrogate marker for AUC when multiple serum vancomycin concentrations are not available to determine the AUC. In this sense, current recommendations have increased the so-called therapeutic range for trough levels from 5-10 mg/L to 10-15 mg/L and 15-20 mg/L, depending on the nature of the infection to be treated.

Keywords: Vancomycin, *Staphyloccocus aureus*, toxicity, pharmacokinetics, pharmacodynamics, therapeutic drug monitoring

Introduction

Vancomycin was first discovered in the 1950s by Eli Lilly and Company. In the early 1950s, the increase of antibiotic-resistant strains of *Staphylococcus aureus* in hospitalized patients with infection prompted a screening program aimed at the development of an effective new agent. In 1952, a missionary in Borneo sent a sample of soil to Edmund Kornfeld, an organic chemist at Eli Lilly. A microorganism (*Streptomyces orientalis*) producing a substance active against gram-positive microorganisms was isolated from that sample, and the active substance, initially referenced as "compound 05865", was eventually given the generic name vancomycin (from the word "vanquish").

The original preparations of vancomycin from fermentation broth contained a number of impurities, and, because of the brown color of the material, it was nicknamed "Mississippi mud" by scientists at Eli Lilly [1]. Vancomycin was not widely used in the two decades following its discovery, in part because of its ototoxicity and nephrotoxicity (probably related to the presence of impurities rather than a direct effect of vancomycin itself), and in part because methicillin and other penicillins active against *S. aureus* were discovered. However, methicillin-resistant *Staphylococcus aureus* (MRSA) infections emerged as a worldwide hospital problem during the 1970s and this fact stimulated the reevaluation of vancomycin in the late 1970s.

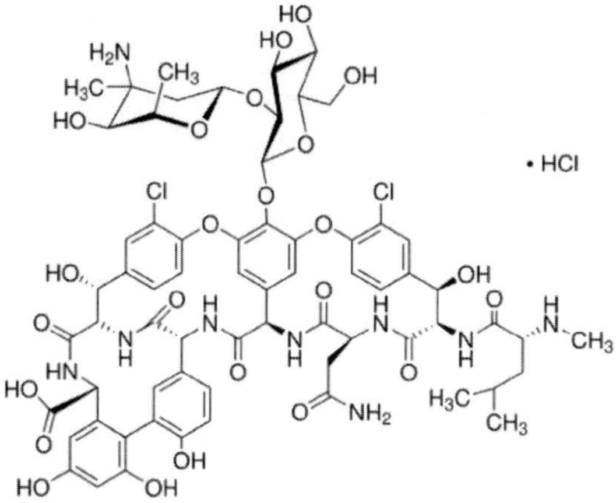

Figure 1. Structural formula of vancomycin hydrocloride.

Newer and purer preparations of vancomycin that produced no ototoxicity and little nephrotoxicity in animal models where obtained, and vancomycin became a key component in the treatment of MRSA infections [1-3]. For over 4 decades, vancomycin has been the antibiotic of choice for infections caused by MRSA. Although newer drugs, such as linezolid and daptomycin, can be as effective as vancomycin in the treatment of some MRSA infections [4-8], vancomycin continues to be the drug of choice for treating most MRSA infections. Vancomycin is a tricyclic glycopeptide antibiotic, with six peptide bonds in its structure and formulated as hydrochloride salt (Figure 1). Vancomycin hydrochloride is highly soluble in water (> 100 mg/mL), moderately soluble in dilute ethanol and insoluble in higher alcohols, acetone or ethers, being -1.44 the calculated log P [9]. Vancomycin is an amphotheric molecule that can react with acids or bases, and for which 6 pKa values have been reported: 7.75, 8.89 (basic), 2.18, 9.59, 10.4, and 12.0 (acidic) [10].

Indications and Efficacy

Vancomycin is active against staphylococci, streptococci, and other gram-positive bacteria but it is not active against gram-negative bacteria, mycobacteria or fungi [11].

Intravenous vancomycin is indicated for the treatment of [11-14]:

- serious infections caused by susceptible strains of methicillin-resistant (beta-lactam-resistant) staphylococci (MRSA and coagulase-negative staphylococcus),
- infections caused by gram-positive organisms in patients with serious allergies to beta-lactam antimicrobials,
- serious invasive infections caused by *Streptococcus pneumoniae* (e.g. endocarditis, meningitis),
- surgical prophylaxis in patients with serious allergies to beta-lactam antimicrobials.

Oral vancomycin is indicated for the treatment of pseudomembranous enterocolitis caused by *Clostridium difficile* and, occasionally, by *S. aureus* [15, 16].

Skin flora is an important source of microorganisms, being responsible for infections produced as a consequence of surgical interventions. The skin flora responsible for most surgical site infections includes *S. aureus*, coagulase-negative staphylococci, *Propionibacterium acnes*, gram-negative bacilli, micrococci, and diphtheroids [17].

S. aureus is a major cause of endocarditis in adults, followed by streptococcus and enterococcus [18]. In contrast, other skin flora rarely produces endocardial infection, with the exception of *Corynebacterium jeikeium* that causes mechanical prosthetic-valve infection [19]. Vancomycin is used for treatment of staphylococcal endocarditis when penicillins cannot be used due to a severe allergy or MRSA is suspected or proven [20]. The effectiveness of vancomycin has also been documented in other infections caused by staphylococci, including septicemia, bone infections, lower respiratory tract infections, and skin infections [21]. Vancomycin is also effective in the treatment of streptococcal endocarditis caused by *Streptococcus viridians* or *Streptococcus bovis*, and it is recommended in patients allergic to penicillins [22]. In these cases, it is administered alone or in combination with an aminoglycoside [23]. In the case of endocarditis caused by enterococcus, it is also administered in combination with an aminoglycoside [20]. Another endocarditis-producing microorganism, *Corynebacterium jeikeium*, is usually susceptible to this drug and resistant to penicillin agents [19].

With the emergence of beta-lactam antibiotic resistance among strains of *Streptococcus pneumoniae*, vancomycin has claimed a more important role in the treatment of meningitis [24]. In fact, vancomycin plus a third-generation cephalosporin (ceftriaxone or cefotaxime) is the standard initial empirical regimen for known or suspected cases of pneumococcal meningitis [25,26]. Use of dexamethasone as adjunct therapy has proved to reduce mortality and neurologic sequelae in adult patients with pneumococcal meningitis. The rationale for use is derived from experimental animal models of infection, which have shown that the subarachnoid space inflammatory response during bacterial meningitis is a major factor contributing to morbidity and mortality [27]. However, use of dexamethasone may impair the penetration of vancomycin in cerebrospinal fluid [28].

Orally administered vancomycin can be used in the treatment of pseudomembranous enterocolitis caused by *Clostridium difficile* and, occasionally, by *S. aureus* [15, 16]. In some clinical studies, equivalent efficacy of metronidazole and vancomycin in mild to moderate *Clostridium difficile* infection [29, 30] has been demonstrated, and some clinical guidelines recomend the use of metronidazole over vancomycin in these cases, taking economic and ecological criteria into account [31-33]. However, other trials have shown the superiority of vancomycin therapy in severely affected patients [34, 35].

Toxicity

Many of the early toxicities observed in patients dosed with vancomycin were attributed to impurities present in preparations elaborated before the mid-1980s [36, 37].

An uncommon infusion-related reaction associated with vancomycin administration is the 'red man' syndrome [38], characterized by flushing of the upper body and pruritus due to histamine release. In some cases, patients with this syndrome also show chest pain, hypotension and muscle spasms [39-41]. The 'red man' syndrome is associated with rapid infusions of vancomycin and it usually occurs within a few minutes after the start of the infusion. Nevertheless, it usually resolves soon after cessation of the infusion and is rarely life-threatening [42, 43].

Adverse effects of vancomycin to the hematopoietic system, such as pancytopenia [44], neutropenia [45, 46] and thrombocytopenia [47-51] are fairly uncommon. Vancomycin-induced neutropenia is relatively rare and is more likely to develop when the drug is administered for > 2 weeks [45, 46]. The mechanism is unknown but thought to be immune-mediated. It appears that neutropenia is not dose- or serum concentration–related, and its incidence is similar across genders and age groups. The majority of cases reported usually resolve within several days of discontinuing vancomycin and the use an alternative antibiotic to complete therapy is generally recommended when possible.

Vancomycin was first associated with thrombocytopenia in 1985 [47]. This was confirmed by further case reports [48-50] and, recently, the clinical course of over 30 patients who developed thrombocytopenia and had vancomycin-dependent anti-platelet antibodies has provided an extensive description of this disorder [51].

Other related side-effects include fixed drug eruptions, fever and phlebitis [52, 53]. A very uncommon vancomycin side effect is the Stevens-Johnson syndrome [54, 55], an acute mucocutaneous process characterized by severe exfoliative dermatitis and mucosal involvement of the gastrointestinal tract and conjunctiva. Treatment of the Stevens-Johnson syndrome consists of cessation of vancomycin and administration of an antihistamine alone or associated with steroid agents [54].

The most commonly described side-effects of vancomycin during the early use of the antibiotic were nephrotoxicity and ototoxicity [56, 57]. However, the incidence of these side-effects related to the use of modern preparations of vancomycin remains controversial.

Although earlier reports on vancomycin nephrotoxicity may have been related to impurities in the product, several studies have shown an association between higher trough concentrations (> 15 mg/L) and nephrotoxicity. Nevertheless, it is generally unclear whether vancomycin is the cause or merely an indicator of renal toxicity [58-60]. Fortunately, vancomycin-related nephrotoxicity is usually reversible, with a low incidence of residual damage if the use of the antibiotic is discontinued or if doses are correctly adjusted immediately after the occurrence of renal failure [60]. There are many different risk factors which could accelerate or potentiate the occurrence of vancomycin nephrotoxicity.

The most highly documented risk factors are (1) high trough vancomycin level (especially > 20 mg/L) or doses (> 4 g/day); (2) treatment with concomitant nephrotoxic agents, such as aminoglycosides; (3) prolonged therapy (more than 7 days); (4), admittance to an intensive care unit (especially long-term stays).

Less commonly mentioned risk factors are advanced age, intermittent dosing, high peak vancomycin level, male sex, vascular surgery, baseline high serum creatinine (> 1.7 mg/dl), peritonitis, liver disease, cancer and neutropenia, furosemide therapy, high APACHE III score, weight of > 101 kg and presence of decubitus ulcer [61].

The overall incidence of ototoxicity associated to vancomycin appears to be low [62].

In 1958, Geraci et al [63] described two cases of irreversible ototoxicity secondary to vancomycin therapy, with serum concentrations ranging from 80 to 100 mg/L. However, the impurities present in these early preparations of vancomycin might have been responsible, at least in part, for such toxicity [37].

Ototoxicity secondary to vancomycin is characterized as damage to the auditory nerve that initially affects high-frequency sensory hairs in the cochlea, then the middle- and low-frequency hairs, and eventually can lead to total hearing loss [37].

High-tone deafness occurs before low-tone deafness at all frequencies and is permanent. Inability to hear high-frequency sounds and tinnitus are ominous signs that should result in discontinuation of vancomycin [64]. Reversible ototoxicity, such as tinnitus, is also rare and may occur with or without high-tone deafness [65, 66].

In 1994, Saunders et al [67] indicated that reversible ototoxicity was generally associated with concentrations > 40 mg/L, and that irreversible damage was a rare complication of vancomycin therapy, encountered in patients with concentrations > 80 mg/L and preexisting renal impairment. Nevertheless, the relationship between vancomycin levels and ototoxicity has not been clearly established and remains controversial [37, 68].

Drug Interactions

Vancomycin is a drug with minimal drug interactions. The most important drug interactions are pharmacodynamic, not pharmacokinetic, in nature [12].

Coadministration of aminoglucoside antibiotics enhances the nephrotoxicity potential of vancomycin [69, 70], and serum creatinine concentrations should be monitored on a daily basis. Vancomycin nephrotoxicity may result from coadministration with tenofovir, a nephrotoxic agent that may increase the risk and severity of renal failure along prolonged vancomycin administration [71].

Vancomycin may increase the risk of bleeding in patients receiving warfarin [72], and it has been indicated that the prothrombin time ratio should be monitored in patients receiving both drugs [12].

Analytical Methods

Vancomycin concentration in biologic fluids has been determined by high-performance liquid chromatography (HPLC, Table 1) [73-82], radioimmunoassay (RIA) [83], enzyme multiplied immunoassay technique (EMIT) [84, 85], microbiologic techniques [86], or fluorescence polarization immunoassay (FPIA) [81, 82, 87].

Fluorescence polarization immunoassay (FPIA) is popular because of its convenience and high throughput capability. However, FPIA requires expensive devices and reagents. The EMIT assay shows improved specificity, but is less precise and less sensitive.

Pharmacokinetics and Pharmacodynamics

The vancomycin serum concentration vs time profile obtained after intravenous administration is polyexponential and has been described with one-, two-, and three-compartment pharmacokinetic models. After the distribution phase(s), a linear (one-exponential) postdistribution phase is obtained with a terminal half-life of 6-12 hours in adult patients with normal renal function [57]. The volume of distribution ranges from 0.4 to 1 L/kg [10], and mean clearance is about 0.06 L/h/kg [88, 89].

Vancomycin absorption from the gastrointestinal tract is negligible. However, some systemic absorption of orally administered vancomycin has been observed in individuals with inflamed colonic mucosa, for example, in patients with pseudomembranous colitis [90-94]. Vancomycin is very irritating to tissue [95] and causes injection site necrosis if injected intramuscularly.

The mean protein binding of vancomycin reported in the literature is 46% [95-99]. Vancomycin distributes into most body spaces, but the concentrations obtained are highly variable and affected by inflammation and disease state. The penetration of vancomycin into the cerebrospinal fluid (CSF) of patients with uninflamed meninges is limited, and low concentrations ranging from 0 to approximately 4 mg/L have been reported, with corresponding CSF-to-serum ratios of 0-0.18, whereas concentrations of 6.4-11.1 mg/L, and CSF-to-serum ratios of 0.36-0.48, have been reported in the presence of inflammation [57, 100, 101]. Vancomycin concentrations in lung tissue ranging from 5% to 41% of serum vancomycin concentrations have been reported in studies of healthy volunteers and patients [57].

Table 1. Summary of HPLC methods for quantification of vancomycin in biological fluids

Matrix	Sample pretreatment	Column	Mobile phase	LOQ (ng/ml)	LOD (ng/ml)	Detection	Ref.
Human plasma and serum	LLE with a 1:1 mixture of hexane:MTBE	Microsorb-MV NH$_2$ (250 x 4.6 mm, 5μm)	*Isocratic* ACN:0.02M phosphate buffer (pH 7) (62:38, v/v), Flow = 2 ml/min	*na*	320	UV (225 nm)	[73]
Human plasma	PP with PCA and LE with DCM	Nucleosil RP-18 (150 x 4.6 mm, 5 μm), 30 °C	*Isocratic* 0.005M KH$_2$PO$_4$ (pH 2.8):ACN (90:10, v/v) Flow = 1.0 ml/min	1000	200	UV (229 nm)	[74]
Human plasma and serum	Dissolution in DMF:H$_2$O (2:3, v:v)	Waters Bondapak C$_{18}$ (300 x 3.9 mm)	*Gradient* MPA = 50 mM ammonium acetate MPB = ACN Flow = 1.5 ml/min	*na*	*na*	UV (230 nm)	[81]
Human serum	SPE	YMC Pack ODS-AQ C$_{18}$ (250 x 4.6 mm, 5 μm)	*Gradient* MPA = 0.05 M buffer phosphate (pH 6):ACN: MeOH (91:5:4, v/v/v) MPB = 0.05 M buffer phosphate (pH6):ACN: MeOH (84:8:8, v/v/v) Flow = 1.5 ml/min	1000	*na*	UV (210 nm)	[75]
Human plasma, tissue and bone samples	SPE	Hypersil BDS C$_8$ (10 cm x 4.6 mm, 3 μm) (23–25°C)	*Gradient* MPA = 5 mM KH$_2$PO$_4$ (pH 2.8) MPB = ACN Flow = 1.5 ml/min	500	*na*	UV (282 nm)	[82]
Human serum	Direct serum injection	Octyl-C$_8$ silica (150 x4.6 mm, 5 μm), 25° C	*Isocratic* 0.1 M phosphate buffer: ACN (95:5, v/v), (pH 7.0) Flow = 0.8 ml/min	*na*	500	UV (240 nm)	[76]

Table 1. (Continued)

Matrix	Sample pretreatment	Column	Mobile phase	LOQ (ng/ml)	LOD (ng/ml)	Detection	Ref.
Human plasma	LLE with MeOH	Kromasil C$_{18}$ (250 x 4.6 mm, 5 μm)	*Isocratic* ACN:25 mM phosphate buffer (pH 7) (12:88, v/v), Flow = 0.8 ml/min	1000	500	UV (215 nm) ED (+700 mV)	[77]
Human serum	Direct serum injection	Octyl-C$_8$ silica (150 x 4.6 mm, 5 μm), 25° C	*Isocratic* 0.1 M phosphate buffer: ACN (95:5, v/v), (pH 7.0) Flow = 0.8 ml/min	1000	1000	UV (240 nm)	[78]
Human plasma	PP with MOPS and ACN	Sulpelcosil LC-18 (250 x 4.6 mm, 5 μm), 25° C	*Isocratic* 75 mM acetate buffer:ACN (92:8, v/v) (pH 5.0) Flow = 0.8 ml/min	400	200	UV (230 nm)	[79]
Human plasma	LLE with EA	Zorbax Eclipse XDB-C8 (125 × 4.0 mm; 5 μm), 30°C	*Gradient* MPA = MeOH MPB = 0.1 M Na2HPO$_4$ (40:60, v:v) Flow = 1 ml/min	*na*	*na*	DAD (200 - 380 nm)	[80]

ACN: acetonitrile; DAD: diode array detector; DCM: dichloromethane; DMF: dimethylformamide; EA: ethyl acetate; ED: electrochemical; LLE: liquid-liquid extraction; LOD: limit of detection; LOQ: limit of quantification; MeOH: methanol; MOPS: 3-[N-morpholino]propanesulfonic acid; MPA: mobile phase A; MPB: mobile phase B; MTBE: methyl tert-butyl ether; *na*: not available. PCA: perchloric acid; PP: protein precipitation; SPE: solid-phase extraction; UV: ultraviolet.

In a study on the penetration of vancomycin in bones of patients undergoing total hip arthroplasty and having vancomycin (15 mg/kg intravenously) administered 1 h prior to anesthesia, it was observed that the vancomycin levels in bones were, in most patients, higher than the minimum inhibitory concentration (MIC) for susceptible staphylococci [102]. However, in the case of patients with osteomyelitis who received doses adjusted to achieve peak levels in serum of 20 to 30 mg/L and trough levels of less than 12 mg/L, the penetration of the antibiotic into bone was variable and the authors suggested additional studies [102]. In another study vancomycin was given for prophylasis during cardiac operations, and the concentrations of the antibiotic in the sternal bone of patients represented 30 to 70% of the concentration in plasma, with a mean bone concentration of 9.3 μg/g.

According to the authors, the concentrations of vancomycin in sternal bones were always above the MICs for staphylococci, streptococci, and enteococci [103].

Skhirtladze et al. [104] measured vancomycin concentrations in the interstitium of soft tissue by means of a microdialysis probe inserted at the thigh of diabetic and nondiabetic patients. In nondiabetic patients, vancomycin tissue-to-plasma concentration ratio was 0.3 and the median tissue concentration was 11.9 mg/L, whereas in the group of diabetic patients, the tissue-to-plama ratio was 0.1 and the median tissue concentration was 3.7 mg/L. The authors concluded that vancomycin penetration into target tissues is substantially impaired in diabetic patients versus nondiabetics, and that the insufficient tissue concentrations could therefore possibly contribute to failure of antibiotic treatment and the development of antimicrobial resistance in diabetic patients.

Most of the administered dose of vancomycin is excreted unchanged in urine within 24 hours after administration [105] by glomerular filtration [106], although small amounts of tubular vancomycin transport cannot be excluded [106, 107]. In healthy subjects, about 30% of the systemic vancomycin clearance is by nonrenal mechanisms, and this nonrenal clearance is concentration-dependent [106].

Pharmacodynamics correlates the concentration of a drug with its pharmacological or clinical effects. For an antibiotic, this correlation refers to the drug concentration and its ability to kill or inhibit the growth of microorganisms. The primary measure of antibiotic activity is the MIC, which is the lowest concentration of an antibiotic that completely inhibits the growth of a microorganism in vitro. However, it does not indicate anything concerning the time course of antimicrobial activity, which can be obtained by means of an integration between pharmacokinetics and pharmacodynamics.

Vancomycin is a time-dependent (concentration-independent) killer of gram-positive pathogens, and several pharmacokinetic and pharmacodynamic monitoring parameters have been proposed for predicting the effectiveness of a given vancomycin regimen: the time the drug concentration remains above the MIC (t > MIC), the maximum serum drug concentration to MIC ratio (C_{max}/MIC), and the area under the serum drug concentration-versus-time curve to MIC ratio (AUC/MIC). At present, the AUC/MIC ratio is the preferred monitoring parameter, and a ratio of $\geq$ 400 has been advocated as a target to achieve clinical effectiveness [57].

The susceptibility and resistance breakpoints for the MIC of vancomycin against S. aureus have been established [108] at $\leq$ 2 mg/L (susceptible), 4-8 mg/L (intermediate), and $\geq$ 16 mg/L (resistant). In addition to these two categories of non-susceptible *S. aureus* (vancomycin intermediate *S. aureus* (VISA) and vancomycin resistant *S. aureus* (VRSA), another category, named "heteroresistant vancomycin intermediate *S. aureus*" (hVISA), is used to describe strains of *S. aureus* that appear to be susceptible to vancomycin by standard broth microdilution techniques but contain subpopulations of vancomycin intermediate cells (detected with BHI screening agar) [109].

Dosing

In general, vancomycin dosing guidelines recommend an initial dosage based on actual body weight and renal function [57, 110]. Vancomycin is usually administered by means of intermittent intravenous infusions, at a rate not exceeding 10 mg/min or over a period of time of at least 60 minutes (to prevent the "red man syndrome"). In adults with normal renal function, the usual intravenous dose is 30 mg/kg/d administered in two divided doses [12], and a loading dose of 25–30 mg/kg (based on actual body weight) can be used in seriously ill patients [57]. The daily dose for obese patients (> 30 % over ideal body weight) is calculated based on the total body weight, but a dosing interval of 8 hours is required to maintain therapeutic trough concentrations given the shorter half-life of vancomycin in these patients [12]. The recommended initial doses for critically ill patients with acute renal failure undergoing continuous hemofiltration (CVVH) are a loading dose of 15-20 mg/kg followed by 250-500 mg every 12 hours [111]. For patients undergoing continuous ateriovenus hemofiltration (CAVH), the recommended initial dose is 500 mg every 24-48 hours [112]. Vancomycin is eliminated principally by glomerular filtration and, therefore, renal dysfunction has a high influence on vancomycin pharmacokinetics [113, 114]. In fact, vancomycin total clearance decreases proportionally to decreases in creatinine clearance [113] and this has lead to the development of nomograms for the initial dosing of vancomycin in adults, taking into account the renal function of the patient estimated through creatinine clearance [113, 114]. The Moellering nomogram [113] was designed to achieve an average steady-state vancomycin concentration of 15 mg/L, whereas the Matzke nomogram [114] was designed to obtain steady-state vancomycin concentrations of 30 mg/L (peak) and 7.5 mg/L (trough).

Intravenous doses for neonates, infants and children with normal renal function are different from doses used in adults. In the case of neonates, intravenous doses are based on birthweigtht and postnatal age [12, 115] (Table 2) or actual weight and postmenstrual age [116].

Table 2. Intravenous doses for neonates based on weight and postnatal age [12]

Weight	< 7 days	≥ 7 days
< 1.2 kg	15 mg/kg every 24 hours	15 mg/kg every 24 hours
1.2-2 kg	10-15 mg/kg every 12-18 hours	10-15 mg/kg every 8-12 hours
> 2 kg	10-15 mg/kg every 8-12 hours	10-15 mg/kg every 6-8 hours

Intravenous doses for infants (over 1 month) and children are 60 mg/kg/d given every 6 hours for central nervous system infections, 40-60 mg/kg/d given every 6 hours for severe infections, and 40 mg/kg/d given every 6-8 hours for other infections with a maximum of 1 g/dose [12].

Orally administered vancomycin can be used in *Clostridium difficile* infection. The common dose administered in adults is 125 mg every 6 hours for an average of 10 days (a higher dose may be considered if the infection fails to respond or if it is severe) [15]. Vancomycin should not be given orally for systemic infections since it is not significantly absorbed.

Therapeutic Drug Monitoring

Therapeutic drug monitoring of vancomycin is frequently used to decrease incidence of toxicity and to improve the therapeutic effect. Due to the interindividual variability of the pharmacokinetic parameters of vancomycin, doses calculated using patient characteristics will not always produce the expected vancomycin serum concentrations.

Circumstances in which therapeutic drug monitoring (TDM) is warranted include: patients receiving concomitant aminoglycoside therapy, patients receiving higher than normal doses of vancomycin (i.e., for meningitis), patients with (potentially) altered pharmacokinetic parameters (pregnant women, burn, trauma and obese patients), patients on haemodialysis, and patients with impaired renal function [68, 117-119].

Over the years, serum vancomycin concentrations monitoring practices have varied. Early suggestions recommended peak serum vancomycin concentrations of 30-40 mg/L and trough concentrations of 5-10 mg/L [120]. However, the most recent recommended monitoring parameter is the AUC to

MIC ratio, which has been found to correlate with efficacy in experiments conducted with in vitro or animal models [57, 101]. However, because it can be difficult in the clinical setting to obtain enough serum vancomycin concentrations to accurately calculate the AUC/MIC ratio, the though serum vancomycin concentration is used as a surrogate marker for AUC [57]. Therefore, trough serum vancomycin concentrations are the most accurate and practical method for monitoring vancomycin effectiveness, and it is recommended that trough serum vancomycin concentrations always be maintained above 10 mg/L to avoid development of resistance [57], and above 15 mg/L in the case of complicated MRSA infections [12, 57]. However, the vancomycin trough serum concentration should not be higher than 20 mg/L in order to prevent vancomycin-associated toxicities.

Conclusion

Vancomycin has been the antibiotic of choice for infections caused by MRSA for over 4 decades. Although newer drugs can be as effective as vancomycin in the treatment of some MRSA infections, vancomycin continues to be the drug of choice for treating most MRSA infections. The initial dosing of vancomycin is influenced by age, body weight renal function and specific pathologies of patients. Subsequent dosing should be adjusted based on serum vancomycin levels, using the AUC/MIC ratio as target (AUC/MIC ≥ 400), or trough concentrations as a surrogate marker for AUC. The recommended through levels are 10-15 mg/L or 15-20 mg/L, depending on the nature of the infection to be treated.

Acknowledgments

Iris Usach is recipient of a predoctoral fellowship from the "Atracció de Talent, VLC-CAMPUS" program of the University of Valencia.

References

[1]   Moellering, R. C. Jr. Vancomycin: a 50-year reassessment. *Clin. Infect. Dis.* 2006 Jan 1; 42 Suppl 1:S3-4.

[2]   Griffith, R. S. Vancomycin use--an historical review. *J. Antimicrob. Chemother.* 1984 Dec; 14 Suppl D:1-5.

[3]   Levine, D. P. Vancomycin: a history. *Clin. Infect. Dis.* 2006 Jan 1; 42 Suppl 1:S5-12.

[4]   Hidron, A. I.; Kempker, R.; Moanna, A.; Rimland, D. Methicillin-resistant Staphylococcus aureus in HIV-infected patients. *Infect. Drug Resist.* 2010; 3:73-86.

[5]   Caffrey, A. R.; Quilliam, B. J.; LaPlante, K. L. Comparative effectiveness of linezolid and vancomycin among a national cohort of patients infected with methicillin-resistant Staphylococcus aureus. *Antimicrob. Agents Chemother.* 2010 Oct; 54(10): 4394-4400.

[6]   Pletz, M. W.; Burkhardt, O.; Welte, T. Nosocomial methicillin-resistant Staphylococcus aureus (MRSA) pneumonia: linezolid or vancomycin? - Comparison of pharmacology and clinical efficacy. *Eur. J. Med. Res.* 2010 Nov 30; 15(12):507-513.

[7]   Walkey, A. J.; O'Donnell, M. R.; Wiener, R. S. Linezolid vs glycopeptide antibiotics for the treatment of suspected methicillin-resistant Staphylococcus aureus nosocomial pneumonia: a meta-analysis of randomized controlled trials. *Chest* 2011 May; 139(5): 1148-1155.

[8]   Wunderink, R. G.; Niederman, M. S.; Kollef, M. H.; Shorr, A. F.; Kunkel, M. J.; Baruch, A. et al. Linezolid in methicillin-resistant Staphylococcus aureus nosocomial pneumonia: a randomized, controlled study. *Clin. Infect. Dis.* 2012 Mar 1; 54(5): 621-629.

[9]   Domenech, O.; Francius, G.; Tulkens, P. M.; Van Bambeke, F.; Dufrene, Y.; Mingeot-Leclercq, M. P. Interactions of oritavancin, a new lipoglycopeptide derived from vancomycin, with phospholipid bilayers: Effect on membrane permeability and nanoscale lipid membrane organization. *Biochim. Biophys. Acta* 2009 Sep; 1788(9): 1832-1840.

[10]   Johnson, J. L.; Yalkowsky, S. H. Reformulation of a new vancomycin analog: an example of the importance of buffer species and strength. *AAPS Pharm. Sci. Tech.* 2006 Jan 13; 7(1):E5.

[11]   Avent, M. L.; Vaska, V. L.; Rogers, B. A.; Cheng, A. C.; van Hal, S. J.; Holmes, N. E. et al. Vancomycin therapeutics and monitoring: a contemporary approach. *Intern. Med. J.* 2013 Feb; 43(2): 110-119.

[12]   Bauer, L. Vancomycin. *Applied Clinical Pharmacokinetics.* 2nd ed ed. New York: McGraw Hill Medical; 2008. p. 207-298.

[13]   Bratzler, D. W.; Dellinger, E. P.; Olsen, K. M.; Perl, T. M.; Auwaerter, P. G.; Bolon, M. K. et al. Clinical practice guidelines for antimicrobial

prophylaxis in surgery. *Am. J. Health Syst. Pharm.* 2013 Feb 1; 70(3): 195-283.

[14] Taubert, K. A.; Dajani, A. S. Preventing bacterial endocarditis: American Heart Association guidelines. *Am. Fam. Physician* 1998 Feb 1; 57(3): 457-468.

[15] Fekety, R.; Silva, J.; Kauffman, C.; Buggy, B.; Deery, H. G. Treatment of antibiotic-associated Clostridium difficile colitis with oral vancomycin: comparison of two dosage regimens. *Am. J. Med.* 1989 Jan; 86(1): 15-19.

[16] Gravet, A.; Rondeau, M.; Harf-Monteil, C.; Grunenberger, F.; Monteil, H.; Scheftel, J. M. et al. Predominant Staphylococcus aureus isolated from antibiotic-associated diarrhea is clinically relevant and produces enterotoxin A and the bicomponent toxin LukE-lukD. *J. Clin. Microbiol.* 1999 Dec; 37(12): 4012-4019.

[17] Dohmen, P. M. Influence of skin flora and preventive measures on surgical site infection during cardiac surgery. *Surg. Infect.* (Larchmt) 2006; 7 Suppl 1:S13-7.

[18] Martinez-Marcos, F. J.; Lomas-Cabezas, J. M.; Hidalgo-Tenorio, C.; de la Torre-Lima, J.; Plata-Ciezar, A.; Reguera-Iglesias, J. M. et al. Enterococcal endocarditis: a multicenter study of 76 cases. *Enferm. Infecc. Microbiol. Clin.* 2009 Dec; 27(10): 571-579.

[19] Mookadam, F.; Cikes, M.; Baddour, L. M.; Tleyjeh, I. M.; Mookadam, M. Corynebacterium jeikeium endocarditis: a systematic overview spanning four decades. *Eur. J. Clin. Microbiol. Infect. Dis.* 2006 Jun; 25(6): 349-353.

[20] Elliott, T. S.; Foweraker, J.; Gould, F. K.; Perry, J. D.; Sandoe, J. A. Working Party of the British Society for Antimicrobial Chemotherapy. Guidelines for the antibiotic treatment of endocarditis in adults: report of the Working Party of the British Society for Antimicrobial Chemotherapy. *J. Antimicrob. Chemother.* 2004 Dec; 54(6): 971-981.

[21] Estes, K. S.; Derendorf, H. Comparison of the pharmacokinetic properties of vancomycin, linezolid, tigecyclin, and daptomycin. *Eur. J. Med. Res.* 2010 Nov 30; 15(12): 533-543.

[22] Martinez, F.; Martin Luengo, F.; Valdes, M. Treatment with vancomycin of experimental endocarditis caused by Streptococcus sanguis II resistant to penicillin. *Enferm. Infecc. Microbiol. Clin.* 1993 May; 11(5): 255-259.

[23] Besnier, J. M.; Leport, C.; Bure, A.; Vilde, J. L. Vancomycin-aminoglycoside combinations in therapy of endocarditis caused by

Enterococcus species and Streptococcus bovis. *Eur. J. Clin. Microbiol. Infect. Dis.* 1990 Feb; 9(2): 130-133.

[24] Ahmed, A. A critical evaluation of vancomycin for treatment of bacterial meningitis. *Pediatr. Infect. Dis. J.* 1997 Sep; 16(9): 895-903.

[25] Tunkel, A. R. Hartman BJ, Kaplan SL, Kaufman BA, Roos KL, Scheld WM, et al. Practice guidelines for the management of bacterial meningitis. *Clin. Infect. Dis.* 2004 Nov 1; 39(9): 1267-1284.

[26] van de Beek, D.; de Gans, J.; Tunkel, A. R.; Wijdicks, E. F. Community-acquired bacterial meningitis in adults. *N. Engl. J. Med.* 2006 Jan 5; 354(1): 44-53.

[27] Tunkel, A. *Bacterial meningitis*. Philadelphia: Lippincott Williams & Wilkins; 2001.

[28] Ricard, J. D.; Wolff, M.; Lacherade, J. C.; Mourvillier, B.; Hidri, N.; Barnaud, G. et al. Levels of vancomycin in cerebrospinal fluid of adult patients receiving adjunctive corticosteroids to treat pneumococcal meningitis: a prospective multicenter observational study. *Clin. Infect. Dis.* 2007 Jan 15; 44(2): 250-255.

[29] Teasley, D. G.; Gerding, D. N.; Olson, M. M.; Peterson, L. R.; Gebhard, R. L.; Schwartz, M. et al. Prospective randomised trial of metronidazole versus vancomycin for Clostridium-difficile-associated diarrhoea and colitis. *Lancet* 1983 Nov 5; 2(8358): 1043-1046.

[30] Wenisch, C.; Parschalk, B.; Hasenhundl, M.; Hirschl, A. M.; Graninger, W. Comparison of vancomycin, teicoplanin, metronidazole, and fusidic acid for the treatment of Clostridium difficile-associated diarrhea. *Clin. Infect. Dis.* 1996 May; 22(5): 813-818.

[31] Cohen, S. H.; Gerding, D. N.; Johnson, S.; Kelly, C. P.; Loo, V. G.; McDonald, L. C. et al. Clinical practice guidelines for Clostridium difficile infection in adults: 2010 update by the society for healthcare epidemiology of America (SHEA) and the infectious diseases society of America (IDSA). *Infect. Control Hosp. Epidemiol.* 2010 May; 31(5): 431-455.

[32] Bauer, T. M.; Lalvani, A.; Fehrenbach, J.; Steffen, I.; Aponte, J. J.; Segovia, R. et al. Derivation and validation of guidelines for stool cultures for enteropathogenic bacteria other than Clostridium difficile in hospitalized adults. *JAMA* 2001 Jan 17; 285(3): 313-319.

[33] McCollum, D. L.; Rodriguez, J. M. Detection, treatment, and prevention of Clostridium difficile infection. *Clin. Gastroenterol. Hepatol.* 2012 Jun; 10(6): 581-592.

[34] Zar, F. A.; Bakkanagari, S. R.; Moorthi, K. M.; Davis, M. B. A comparison of vancomycin and metronidazole for the treatment of Clostridium difficile-associated diarrhea, stratified by disease severity. *Clin. Infect. Dis.* 2007 Aug 1; 45(3): 302-307.

[35] Louie, T.; Gerdsom, M.; Grimard, D. Results of a phase III trial comparing tolevamer, vancomicin and metronidazole in Clostridium difficile associated diarrhea (CDAD) [abstract K-425a]. *47th Interscience Conference on Antimicrobial Agents and Chemotherapy;* September 17 - 20, 2007; Chicago, USA.

[36] Hodoshima, N.; Masuda, S.; Inui, K. Decreased renal accumulation and toxicity of a new VCM formulation in rats with chronic renal failure. *Drug Metab. Pharmacokinet.* 2007 Dec; 22(6): 419-427.

[37] Bailie, G. R.; Neal, D. Vancomycin ototoxicity and nephrotoxicity. A review. *Med. Toxicol. Adverse Drug Exp.* 1988 Sep-Oct; 3(5): 376-386.

[38] Davis, R. L.; Smith, A. L.; Koup, J. R. The Red Man's Syndrome and Slow Infusion of Vancomycin. *Ann. Intern. Med.* 1986; 104(2): 285-286.

[39] Garrelts, J. C.; Peterie, J. D. Vancomycin and the "red man's syndrome". *N. Engl. J. Med.* 1985 Jan 24; 312(4): 245.

[40] Cole, D. R.; Oliver, M.; Coward, R. A.; Brown, C. B. Allergy, red man syndrome, and vancomycin. *Lancet* 1985 Aug 3; 2(8449): 280.

[41] Wallace, M. R.; Mascola, J. R.; Oldfield, E. C. 3rd. Red man syndrome: incidence, etiology, and prophylaxis. *J. Infect. Dis.* 1991 Dec; 164(6): 1180-1185.

[42] Levy, M.; Koren, G.; Dupuis, L.; Read, S. E. Vancomycin-induced red man syndrome. *Pediatrics* 1990 Oct; 86(4): 572-580.

[43] Polk, R. E. Red man syndrome. *Ann. Pharmacother.* 1998 Jul-Aug; 32(7-8): 840.

[44] Shahar, A.; Berner, Y.; Levi, S. Fever, rash, and pancytopenia following vancomycin rechallenge in the presence of ceftazidime. *Ann. Pharmacother.* 2000 Feb; 34(2): 263-264.

[45] Farber, B. F.; Moellering, R. C. Jr. Retrospective study of the toxicity of preparations of vancomycin from 1974 to 1981. *Antimicrob. Agents Chemother.* 1983 Jan; 23(1): 138-141.

[46] Smith, P. F.; Taylor, C. T. Vancomycin-induced neutropenia associated with fever: similarities between two immune-mediated drug reactions. *Pharmacotherapy* 1999 Feb; 19(2): 240-244.

[47] Walker, R. W.; Heaton, A. Thrombocytopenia due to vancomycin. *Lancet* 1985 Apr 20; 1(8434):932.

[48] Christie, D. J.; van Buren, N.; Lennon, S. S.; Putnam, J. L. Vancomycin-dependent antibodies associated with thrombocytopenia and refractoriness to platelet transfusion in patients with leukemia. *Blood* 1990 Jan 15; 75(2):518-523.

[49] Mizon, P.; Kiefel, V.; Mannessier, L.; Mueller-Eckhardt, C.; Goudemand, J. Thrombocytopenia induced by vancomycin-dependent platelet antibody. *Vox. Sang.* 1997; 73(1): 49-51.

[50] Kenney, B.; Tormey, C. A. Acute vancomycin-dependent immune thrombocytopenia as an anamnestic response. *Platelets* 2008 Aug; 19(5): 379-383.

[51] Von Drygalski, A.; Curtis, B. R.; Bougie, D. W.; McFarland, J. G.; Ahl, S.; Limbu, I. et al. Vancomycin-induced immune thrombocytopenia. *N. Engl. J. Med.* 2007 Mar 1; 356(9): 904-910.

[52] Woodley, D. W.; Hall, W. H. The treatment of severe staphylococcal infections with vancomycin. *Ann. Intern. Med.* 1961 Aug; 55: 235-249.

[53] Geraci, J. E.; Nichols, D. R.; Wellman, W. E. Vancomycin in serious staphylococcal infections. *Arch. Intern. Med.* 1962 May; 109: 507-515.

[54] Alexander II; Greenberger, P. A. Vancomycin-induced Stevens-Johnson syndrome. *Allergy Asthma Proc.* 1996 Mar-Apr; 17(2): 75-78.

[55] Laurencin, C. T.; Horan, R. F.; Senatus, P. B.; Wheeler, C. B.; Lipson, S. J. Stevens-Johnson-type reaction with vancomycin treatment. *Ann. Pharmacother.* 1992 Dec; 26(12): 1520-1521.

[56] Forouzesh, A.; Moise, P. A.; Sakoulas, G. Vancomycin ototoxicity: a reevaluation in an era of increasing doses. *Antimicrob. Agents Chemother.* 2009 Feb; 53(2): 483-486.

[57] Rybak, M.; Lomaestro, B.; Rotschafer, J. C.; Moellering, R. Jr; Craig, W.; Billeter, M. et al. Therapeutic monitoring of vancomycin in adult patients: a consensus review of the American Society of Health-System Pharmacists, the Infectious Diseases Society of America, and the Society of Infectious Diseases Pharmacists. *Am. J. Health Syst. Pharm.* 2009 Jan 1;66(1): 82-98.

[58] Jeffres, M. N.; Isakow, W.; Doherty, J. A.; Micek, S. T.; Kollef, M. H. A retrospective analysis of possible renal toxicity associated with vancomycin in patients with health care-associated methicillin-resistant Staphylococcus aureus pneumonia. *Clin. Ther.* 2007 Jun; 29(6): 1107-1115.

[59] Hidayat, L. K.; Hsu, D. I.; Quist, R.; Shriner, K. A.; Wong-Beringer, A. High-dose vancomycin therapy for methicillin-resistant Staphylococcus

aureus infections: efficacy and toxicity. *Arch. Intern. Med.* 2006 Oct 23; 166(19): 2138-2144.

[60]   Zimmermann, A. E.; Katona, B. G.; Plaisance, K. I. Association of vancomycin serum concentrations with outcomes in patients with gram-positive bacteremia. *Pharmacotherapy* 1995 Jan-Feb; 15(1):85-91.

[61]   Elyasi, S.; Khalili, H.; Dashti-Khavidaki, S.; Mohammadpour, A. Vancomycin-induced nephrotoxicity: mechanism, incidence, risk factors and special populations. A literature review. *Eur. J. Clin. Pharmacol.* 2012 Sep; 68(9): 1243-1255.

[62]   Elting, L. S.; Rubenstein, E. B.; Kurtin, D.; Rolston, K. V.; Fangtang, J.; Martin, C. G. et al. Mississippi mud in the 1990s: risks and outcomes of vancomycin-associated toxicity in general oncology practice. *Cancer* 1998 Dec 15; 83(12):2597-2607.

[63]   Geraci, J. E.; Heilman, F. R.; Nichols, D. R.; Wellman, W. E. Antibiotic therapy of bacterial endocarditis. VII. Vancomycin for acute micrococcal endocarditis; preliminary report. *Proc. Staff Meet Mayo. Clin.* 1958 Apr 2; 33(7):172-181.

[64]   Fekety, R. Vancomycin. *Med. Clin. North Am.* 1982 Jan; 66(1):175-181.

[65]   Moise-Broder, P. A.; Sakoulas, G.; Eliopoulos, G. M.; Schentag, J. J.; Forrest, A.; Moellering, R. C. Jr. Accessory gene regulator group II polymorphism in methicillin-resistant Staphylococcus aureus is predictive of failure of vancomycin therapy. *Clin. Infect. Dis.* 2004 Jun 15; 38(12): 1700-1705.

[66]   Traber, P. G.; Levine, D. P. Vancomycin Ototoxity in patient with normal renal function. *Ann. Intern. Med.* 1981 Oct; 95(4): 458-460.

[67]   Saunders, N. J. Why monitor peak vancomycin concentrations? *Lancet* 1994 Dec 24-31; 344(8939-8940): 1748-1750.

[68]   Cantu, T. G.; Yamanaka-Yuen, N. A.; Lietman, P. S. Serum vancomycin concentrations: reappraisal of their clinical value. *Clin. Infect. Dis.* 1994 Apr; 18(4): 533-543.

[69]   Pauly, D. J.; Musa, D. M.; Lestico, M. R.; Lindstrom, M. J.; Hetsko, C. M. Risk of nephrotoxicity with combination vancomycin-aminoglycoside antibiotic therapy. *Pharmacotherapy* 1990; 10(6): 378-382.

[70]   Pannu, N.; Nadim, M. K. An overview of drug-induced acute kidney injury. *Crit. Care Med.* 2008 Apr; 36(4 Suppl): S216-23.

[71]   Psevdos, Jr G.; Gonzalez, E.; Sharp, V. Acute renal failure in patients with AIDS on tenofovir while receiving prolonged vancomycin course for osteomyelitis. *AIDS Read* 2009; 19(6): 245-248.

[72] Angaran, D. M.; Dias, V. C.; Arom, K. V.; Northrup, W. F.; Kersten, T. G.; Lindsay, W. G. et al. The comparative influence of prophylactic antibiotics on the prothrombin response to warfarin in the postoperative prosthetic cardiac valve patient. Cefamandole, cefazolin, vancomycin. *Ann. Surg.* 1987 Aug; 206(2): 155-161.

[73] Li, L.; Miles, M. V.; Hall, W.; Carson, S. W. An improved micromethod for vancomycin determination by high-performance liquid chromatography. *Ther. Drug Monit.* 1995; 17(4): 366-370.

[74] Lukša, J.; Marušič, A. Rapid high-performance liquid chromatographic determination of vancomycin in human plasma. *Journal of Chromatography B: Biomedical Sciences and Applications* 1995; 667(2): 277-281.

[75] Backes, D. W.; Aboleneen, H. I.; Simpson, J. A. Quantitation of vancomycin and its crystalline degradation product (CDP-1) in human serum by high performance liquid chromatography. *J. Pharm. Biomed. Anal.* 1998; 16(8): 1281-1288.

[76] Furuta, I.; Kitahashi, T.; Kuroda, T.; Nishio, H.; Oka, C.; Morishima, Y. Rapid serum vancomycin assay by high-performance liquid chromatography using a semipermeable surface packing material column. *Clinica chimica acta* 2000; 301(1):31-39.

[77] Favetta, P.; Guitton, J.; Bleyzac, N.; Dufresne, C.; Bureau, J. New sensitive assay of vancomycin in human plasma using high-performance liquid chromatography and electrochemical detection. *Journal of Chromatography B: Biomedical Sciences and Applications* 2001; 751(2): 377-382.

[78] Kitahashi, T.; Furuta, I. Determination of vancomycin in human serum by micellar electrokinetic capillary chromatography with direct sample injection. *Clinica chimica acta* 2001; 312(1): 221-225.

[79] López, K.; Bertoluci, D. F.; Vicente, K.; Dell'Aquilla, A.; Santos, S. Simultaneous determination of cefepime, vancomycin and imipenem in human plasma of burn patients by high-performance liquid chromatography. *Journal of Chromatography B* 2007; 860(2): 241-245.

[80] Hu, L. Q.; Yin, C. L.; Du, Y. H.; Zeng, Z. P. Simultaneous and Direct Determination of Vancomycin and Cephalexin in Human Plasma by Using HPLC-DAD Coupled with Second-Order Calibration Algorithms. *J. Anal. Methods Chem.* 2012; 2012: 256963.

[81] Adamczyk, M.; Brate, E. M.; Chiappetta, E. G.; Ginsburg, S.; Hoffman, E.; Klein, C. et al. Development of a quantitative vancomycin

immunoassay for the Abbott AxSYM analyzer. *Ther. Drug Monit.* 1998; 20(2): 191-201.

[82] Farin, D.; Piva, G. A.; Gozlan, I.; Kitzes-Cohen, R. A modified HPLC method for the determination of vancomycin in plasma and tissues and comparison to FPIA (TDX). *J. Pharm. Biomed. Anal.* 1998; 18(3): 367-372.

[83] Fong, K.; Ho, D.; Bogerd, L.; Pan, T.; Brown, N.; Gentry, L. et al. Sensitive radioimmunoassay for vancomycin. *Antimicrob. Agents Chemother.* 1981; 19(1): 139-143.

[84] Wilson, J. F.; Davis, A. C.; Tobin, C. M. Evaluation of commercial assays for vancomycin and aminoglycosides in serum: a comparison of accuracy and precision based on external quality assessment. *J. Antimicrob. Chemother.* 2003; 52(1):78-82.

[85] Yeo, K.; Traverse, W.; Horowitz, G. Clinical performance of the EMIT vancomycin assay. *Clin. Chem.* 1989; 35(7): 1504-1507.

[86] Azzazy, H. M.; Chou, P. P.; Tsushima, J. H.; Troxil, S.; Gordon, M.; Avers, R. J. et al. Abbott AxSYM Vancomycin II assay: multicenter evaluation and interference studies. *Ther. Drug Monit.* 1998; 20(2): 202-208.

[87] Filburn, B.; Shull, V.; Tempera, Y.; Dick, J. Evaluation of an automated fluorescence polarization immunoassay for vancomycin. *Antimicrob. Agents Chemother.* 1983; 24(2): 216-220.

[88] Sanchez, J. L.; Dominguez, A. R.; Lane, J. R.; Anderson, P. O.; Capparelli, E. V.; Cornejo-Bravo, J. M. Population pharmacokinetics of vancomycin in adult and geriatric patients: comparison of eleven approaches. *Int. J. Clin. Pharmacol. Ther.* 2010 Aug; 48(8): 525-533.

[89] Yasuhara, M.; Iga, T.; Zenda, H.; Okumura, K.; Oguma, T.; Yano, Y. et al. Population pharmacokinetics of vancomycin in Japanese adult patients. *Ther. Drug Monit.* 1998 Apr; 20(2): 139-148.

[90] Armstrong, C. J.; Wilson, T. S. Systemic absorption of vancomycin. *J. Clin. Pathol.* 1995 Jul; 48(7): 689.

[91] Spitzer, P. G.; Eliopoulos, G. M. Systemic absorption of enteral vancomycin in a patient with pseudomembranous colitis. *Ann. Intern. Med.* 1984 Apr; 100(4): 533-534.

[92] Matzke, G. R.; Halstenson, C. E.; Olson, P. L.; Collins, A. J.; Abraham, P. A. Systemic absorption of oral vancomycin in patients with renal insufficiency and antibiotic-associated colitis. *Am. J. Kidney Dis.* 1987 May; 9(5): 422-425.

[93] Yamazaki, S.; Nakamura, H.; Yamagata, S.; Miura, G.; Hattori, N.; Shinozaki, K. et al. Unexpected serum level of vancomycin after oral administration in a patient with severe colitis and renal insufficiency. Int J. Clin. Pharmacol. Ther. 2009 Nov; 47(11): 701-706.

[94] Aradhyula, S.; Manian, F. A.; Hafidh, S. A.; Bhutto, S. S.; Alpert, M. A. Significant absorption of oral vancomycin in a patient with clostridium difficile colitis and normal renal function. South Med. J. 2006 May; 99(5): 518-520.

[95] Moellering, R. C. Jr, Krogstad, D. J.; Greenblatt, D. J. Pharmacokinetics of vancomycin in normal subjects and in patients with reduced renal function. Rev. Infect. Dis. 1981 Nov-Dec; 3 suppl: S230-5.

[96] Ackerman, B. H.; Taylor, E. H.; Olsen, K. M.; Abdel-Malak, W.; Pappas, A. A. Vancomycin serum protein binding determination by ultrafiltration. Drug Intell. Clin. Pharm. 1988 Apr; 22(4): 300-303.

[97] Albrecht, L. M.; Rybak, M. J.; Warbasse, L. H.; Edwards, D. J. Vancomycin protein binding in patients with infections caused by Staphylococcus aureus. DICP 1991 Jul-Aug; 25(7-8): 713-715.

[98] Bailey, E. M.; Rybak, M. J.; Kaatz, G. W. Comparative effect of protein binding on the killing activities of teicoplanin and vancomycin. Antimicrob. Agents Chemother. 1991 Jun; 35(6):1089-1092.

[99] Butterfield, J. M.; Patel, N.; Pai, M. P.; Rosano, T. G.; Drusano, G. L.; Lodise, T. P. Refining vancomycin protein binding estimates: identification of clinical factors that influence protein binding. Antimicrob. Agents Chemother. 2011 Sep; 55(9): 4277-4282.

[100] Albanese, J.; Leone, M.; Bruguerolle, B.; Ayem, M. L.; Lacarelle, B.; Martin, C. Cerebrospinal fluid penetration and pharmacokinetics of vancomycin administered by continuous infusion to mechanically ventilated patients in an intensive care unit. Antimicrob. Agents Chemother. 2000 May; 44(5): 1356-1358.

[101] Rybak, M. J. The pharmacokinetic and pharmacodynamic properties of vancomycin. Clin. Infect. Dis. 2006 Jan 1; 42 Suppl 1:S35-9.

[102] Graziani, A. L.; Lawson, L. A.; Gibson, G. A.; Steinberg, M. A.; MacGregor, R. R. Vancomycin concentrations in infected and noninfected human bone. Antimicrob. Agents Chemother. 1988 Sep; 32(9): 1320-1322.

[103] Massias, L.; Dubois, C.; de Lentdecker, P.; Brodaty, O.; Fischler, M.; Farinotti, R. Penetration of vancomycin in uninfected sternal bone. Antimicrob. Agents Chemother. 1992 Nov; 36(11): 2539-2541.

[104] Skhirtladze, K.; Hutschala, D.; Fleck, T.; Thalhammer, F.; Ehrlich, M.; Vukovich, T. et al. Impaired target site penetration of vancomycin in diabetic patients following cardiac surgery. *Antimicrob. Agents Chemother.* 2006 Apr; 50(4): 1372-1375.

[105] Matzke, G. R.; Zhanel, G. G.; Guay, D. R. Clinical pharmacokinetics of vancomycin. *Clin. Pharmacokinet.* 1986 Jul-Aug; 11(4):257-282.

[106] Golper, T. A.; Noonan, H. M.; Elzinga, L.; Gilbert, D.; Brummett, R.; Anderson, J. L. et al. Vancomycin pharmacokinetics, renal handling, and nonrenal clearances in normal human subjects. *Clin. Pharmacol. Ther.* 1988 May; 43(5): 565-570.

[107] Fanos, V.; Benini, D.; Vinco, S.; Pizzini, C.; Khoory, B. J. Glycopeptides and the newborn infant's kidney. *Pediatr. Med. Chir.* 1997 Jul-Aug; 19(4): 259-262.

[108] Tenover, F. C.; Moellering, R. C. Jr. The rationale for revising the Clinical and Laboratory Standards Institute vancomycin minimal inhibitory concentration interpretive criteria for Staphylococcus aureus. *Clin. Infect. Dis.* 2007 May 1; 44(9): 1208-1215.

[109] Burnham, C. A.; Weber, C. J.; Dunne, W. M. Jr. Novel screening agar for detection of vancomycin-nonsusceptible Staphylococcus aureus. *J. Clin. Microbiol.* 2010 Mar; 48(3): 949-951.

[110] Liu, C.; Bayer, A.; Cosgrove, S. E.; Daum, R. S.; Fridkin, S. K.; Gorwitz, R. J. et al. Clinical practice guidelines by the infectious diseases society of america for the treatment of methicillin-resistant Staphylococcus aureus infections in adults and children: executive summary. *Clin. Infect. Dis.* 2011 Feb 1; 52(3): 285-292.

[111] Boereboom, F. T.; Ververs, F. F.; Blankestijn, P. J.; Savelkoul, T. J.; van Dijk, A. Vancomycin clearance during continuous venovenous haemofiltration in critically ill patients. *Intensive Care Med.* 1999 Oct; 25(10): 1100-1104.

[112] Gilbert, D.; Moellering, R.; Eliopoulos, G.; Sande, M. The Sanford guide to Antimicrobial Therapy. 37 th ed ed. Sperryville, VA: *Antimicrobial Therapy, Inc.*; 2007.

[113] Moellering, R. C. Jr; Krogstad, D. J.; Greenblatt, D. J. Vancomycin therapy in patients with impaired renal function: a nomogram for dosage. *Ann. Intern. Med.* 1981 Mar; 94(3): 343-346.

[114] Matzke, G. R.; McGory, R. W.; Halstenson, C. E.; Keane, W. F. Pharmacokinetics of vancomycin in patients with various degrees of renal function. *Antimicrob. Agents Chemother.* 1984 Apr; 25(4): 433-437.

[115] Taketomo, C.; Hodding, J.; Kraus, D. *Pediatric dosage handbook*. 2nd edition ed.: Lexi-Comp Inc; 1993.

[116] Marques-Minana, M. R.; Saadeddin, A.; Peris, J. E. Population pharmacokinetic analysis of vancomycin in neonates. A new proposal of initial dosage guideline. *Br. J. Clin. Pharmacol.* 2010 Nov; 70(5): 713-720.

[117] Moellering, R. C. Jr. Monitoring serum vancomycin levels: climbing the mountain because it is there? *Clin. Infect. Dis.* 1994 Apr; 18(4): 544-546.

[118] Karam, C. M.; McKinnon, P. S.; Neuhauser, M. M.; Rybak, M. J. Outcome assessment of minimizing vancomycin monitoring and dosing adjustments. *Pharmacotherapy* 1999 Mar; 19(3): 257-266.

[119] Antibiotic Expert Group. *Therapeutic Guidelines: Antibiotic.* Version 14 ed. Melbourne: Therapeutic Guidelines Limited; 2010.

[120] Geraci, J. E. Vancomycin. *Mayo. Clin. Proc.* 1977 Oct; 52(10): 631-634.

In: Vancomycin   ISBN: 978-1-62948-559-1
Editor: Abu Gafar Hossion   © 2013 Nova Science Publishers, Inc.

Chapter 4

Clinical Use of Vancomycin in Cardiovascular Homograft Banking

Wee Ling Heng[1]*, Yeong Phang Lim[1],
Chong Hee Lim[1] and Linda Manning[2]
[1]National Cardiovascular Homograft Bank,
National Heart Centre Singapore, Singapore
[2]Cell and Tissue Therapies WA, Royal Perth Hospital,
Western Australia

Abstract

Antibiotics are routinely used for the decontamination of cardiovascular homografts. This step of bioburden reduction is critical because manipulation during tissue recovery and processing as well as environmental factors may introduce micro-organisms to the homografts. As the consequences of implanting contaminated homografts are potentially life-threatening, stringent measures are taken to eliminate microbial transmission to recipients. This includes the application of aseptic techniques in tissue recovery and processing as well as antibiotic decontamination of homografts prior to long-term storage in liquid nitrogen vapour.

---

* Corresponding Author: Wee Ling HENG, heng.wee.ling@nhcs.com.sg.

Usually, to target a diverse spectrum of endemic micro-organisms isolated from tissues, a cocktail of different antibiotics are utilised. In 2011, a collation of heart valve processing practices from 24 international heart valve banks in North America, Europe, Australasia and South Africa revealed that vancomycin is one of the most commonly used antibiotics in cardiovascular homograft banking. 62.5% of the banks included vancomycin of concentration 50-500 µg/mL in their antibiotic cocktail. Antibiotic regimens were validated by individual banks prior to implementation to ensure that the antibiotic combination, incubation temperature and condition yielded optimal bactericidal effect. The test systems used to detect microbial contamination of the homografts were also validated to ensure the results were not compromised by the presence of residual antibiotics. At the author's tissue bank, vancomycin is preferred due to its broad spectrum and stability. This article briefly presents findings on the international banks' bioburden reduction practices and discusses the emerging importance of vancomycin in cardiovascular homograft banking.

Keywords: Heart valve banking; tissue banking; cardiovascular homograft banking; microbial contamination; antibiotic decontamination; vancomycin

Introduction

Effective eradication of microbial contamination of homografts is critical to ensure the provision of safe tissue products for implantation. However, procurement of aseptic homografts can be difficult to achieve. Microbial contamination of the homograft can originate from a number of sources, which include the donor, retrieval environment, or even the personnel conducting tissue recovery and processing procedures [1]. For instance, a significantly higher contamination rate of arterial tissues as compared to heart tissues had been reported, which was ascribed to the higher microbial load found in the abdominal compartment where arteries were recovered [2]. Elevated numbers of culture-positive results in homografts from multi-organ donors had also been described. This could occur especially when heart recovery was initiated after organ retrieval team had perforated the bowel or when the heart had been removed with instruments used to recover other tissues. An increase in incidence of contamination had also been reported for valves recovered in open mortuary areas due to reduced air quality of the mortuary environment [3].

Many homografts are recovered from multi-organ donors under conditions that make aseptic retrieval of the tissue difficult or impossible to achieve. Given the potentially life-threatening consequence of implanting a contaminated graft, stringent measures are taken to minimise microbial transmission to recipients as much as possible [4,5,6]. These include adherence to aseptic techniques during tissue retrieval and processing, prompt procurement of tissues after death, reduction in duration of tissue exposure to the retrieval environment, and maintaining separation of the thoracic cavity from the abdominal cavity where possible [3]. Although aseptic procedures are meticulously applied and sterile instruments and materials are used, contamination of recovered homografts cannot be completely eliminated [1].

To address this potential risk to the recipient, dissected homografts undergo a process of bioburden reduction. Although terminal sterilisation by gamma-irradiation can be used for tissues such as bone allografts, soft-tissues such as heart valves cannot be terminally sterilised. It is well recognised that terminal sterilisation of soft-tissues alters the homograft's biomechanical properties [7], inactivates cells within the graft and affects cell viability [8], significantly reducing graft durability and function *in situ*. For these reasons, the majority of heart valve banks worldwide now include a bioburden reduction step using a cocktail of antibiotics during processing to decontaminate homografts prior to long-term storage and implantation.

Bioburden Reduction of Homografts

Previously, decontamination of cardiovascular homografts was conducted using aggressive sterilisation methods, such as gamma-irradiation or chemical disinfection using formaldehyde, glutaraldehyde, beta-propriolactone and ethylene oxide. Although these techniques increased homograft availability, valve durability was adversely affected due to loss of cellular viability and subsequent structural deterioration of the valves [9]. Due to poor clinical outcomes among recipients of these terminally sterilised valves, their use in transplantation declined and remained low for several years. In 1968, Barratt-Boyes et al. developed high-concentration antibiotic decontamination procedures to disinfect heart valves for banking and transplantation [10,11]. These procedures have been refined over the years, with incubation in low-concentration antibiotic solution becoming the most common bioburden reduction method used for disinfecting cardiovascular homografts. Tissues processed using this method were found to maintain their structure, biomechanical properties and cell viability, resulting in improved valve durability and function *in situ*. This outcome led to a revival in the clinical use of homografts for transplantation [3,4,12,13].

Despite the widespread use of antibiotics and its significant impact on successful decontamination of homografts, standardisation of the bioburden reduction step has not been achieved [2,10,13,14,15]. Indeed, a recent survey of 24 heart valve banks identified extensive differences in the composition and concentrations of antibiotics used and in the incubation conditions (durations and temperatures) applied to achieve bioburden reduction [15]. Lack of standardisation of this step is not surprising for a number of reasons. Firstly, banks in different parts of the world contend with different endemic micro-organisms of various antibiotic sensitivities. In addition, some banks have patented the bioburden procedures for their purposes, while others have established protocols that meet their requirements based on experience and outcomes. In all cases, the procedures used had been validated and met the banks' final product requirements.

Emerging Importance of Vancomycin in Tissue Banking

There is a general trend of increasing antibiotic resistance among micro-organisms. For this reason, it is imperative to understand antimicrobial susceptibility patterns of micro-organisms commonly isolated from homografts when choosing an antibiotic combination for the bioburden reduction step. It is well established that the types of microbial contaminants vary with geographical location, and that selection pressures exerted by antibiotic use alters antimicrobial susceptibility patterns. Even so, it has been reported that the susceptibility patterns displayed by micro-organisms isolated from homografts are similar to those found in other clinical circumstances within the same geographical region [6]. This finding provides a rational basis for developing an antibiotic cocktail that will be effective in decontaminating homografts retrieved in the same region.

Vancomycin is a unique glycopeptide structurally unrelated to any currently available antibiotic. Its primary mode of action is achieved by inhibiting bacterial cell wall synthesis of susceptible micro-organisms.

Table 1. Antibiotic regimens of heart valve banks which use vancomycin as one of the antibiotics for decontamination of cardiovascular homografts

Bank	Concentration of vancomycin used	Other antibiotics used	Incubation conditions
Europe: a total of 11 banks surveyed			
E1	500 µg/mL	Gentamicin: 50 µg/mL Piperacillin: 500 µg/mL Nystatin: 2500 U/mL	Room temperature (21°C), 24 hours in the dark
E2	50 µg/mL	Cefoxitin: 240 µg/mL Lincomycin: 120 µg/mL Colimycin: 100 µg/mL	4°C, 24 hours
E3	50 µg/mL	Gentamicin: 4000 µg/mL Imipenem: 200 µg/mL Nystatin: 2500 U/mL Polymixin B: 200 µg/mL	2 - 8°C, 18 - 24 hours
E4	50 µg/mL	Gentamicin: 4000 µg/mL Ciprofloxacin: 200 µg/mL Amphotericin B: 50 µg/mL	Room temperature (21°C), 24 hours
E5	50 µg/mL	Metronidazol: 50 µg/mL Amikacin: 50 µg/mL Amphotericin B: 5 µg/mL	4°C, 24 hours
E6	50 µg/mL	Tobramycin: 50 µg/mL Cotrimoxazole: 50 µg/mL	4°C, 6 - 24 hours
E7	Information not provided	Lincomycin, Polymyxin B sulphate	4°C, 48 hours
E8	500 µg/mL	Amphotericin B: 250 µg/mL Fungoral: 100 µg/mL Colistin: 200 µg/mL Gentamicin: 530 µg/mL	4 - 8°C, 24 hours

Table 1. (Continued)

Bank	Concentration of vancomycin used	Other antibiotics used	Incubation conditions
E9	500 μg/mL	Cefuroxime: 250 μg/mL Gentamicin: 80 μg/mL Ciproflaxacin: 200 μg/mL Colistin: 1000 IU/mL Amphotericin B: 20 μg/mL	37°C, 18 - 24 hours
North America: a total of 6 banks surveyed			
N1	50 μg/mL	Gentamicin: 80 μg/mL Cefoxitin: 240 μg/mL	33 - 38°C, 18 - 26 hours
N2	Information not provided	Cefoxitin, Colymycim-M, Lincomycin	4°C, 24 hours
N3	50 μg/mL	Cefoxitin: 240 μg/mL Polymyxin B: 100 mg/mL Lincomycin: 120 μg/mL	1 - 10°C, 22 - 26 hours
N4	50 μg/mL	Colymycin M: 75 mg/mL Cefoxitin: 100mg/mL Lincomycin: 300 mg/mL	4°C, 24 ± 2 hours
Australasia and South Africa: a total of 7 banks surveyed			
A1	50 μg/mL	Cefoxitin: 240 μg/mL Lincomycin: 120 μg/mL Polymyxin B: 100 μg/mL Amphotericin B: 25 μg/mL	First soak: 4°C, 24 hours; 2nd soak: 4°C, 24 hours; Transfer to Hank's Balanced Salt Solution at 4°C until frozen
A2	50 μg/mL	Amikacin: 100 μg/mL	4°C, 24 - 28 hours

Studies have shown that vancomycin can also alter the permeability of cell membrane and may selectively inhibit ribonucleic acid synthesis [16].

Vancomycin is known to be active against a large number of gram-positive aerobes and anaerobes, such as *Staphylococcus aureus* (including methicillin-resistant strains), *Staphylococcus epidermidis* (including multiple-resistant strains), viridan streptococci, enterococci, and clostridia, amongst others [16,17]. However, it exhibits no significant activity against most gram-negative bacteria, such as *Pseudomonas* species and *Esherichia coli*, which are commonly found in homografts worldwide [17]. Therefore, to cover a wider microbial spectrum, vancomycin must be combined with other antibiotics to effectively reduce microbial load of the homografts.

In 2011, a survey was conducted by co-author Linda Manning to compile information on heart valve processing techniques, including antibiotic regimens, utilised by 24 international heart valve banks from Europe, North America, Australasia and South Africa [15]. As presented in Table 1, results revealed that 62.5% of the banks used vancomycin as one of the antibiotics to decontaminate their homografts. Among the banks that used vancomycin, 60% of them added an aminoglycoside, such as gentamicin, amikacin or tobramycin to the antibiotic mix. Aminoglycosides are preferred because they are bactericidal and active *in-vitro* against a wide spectrum of aerobic and facultative gram-negative bacilli [18]. In addition, the bactericidal activity of vancomycin in combination with an aminoglycoside was found to be synergistic, especially against *Staphylococcus aureus*, enterococci and viridan streptococci [16]. Currently, gentamicin is the aminoglycoside of choice by 66.7% of the banks surveyed using this vancomycin-aminoglycoside combination. This is probably because the combination of vancomycin and gentamicin reportedly yields the most predictable synergistic activity against most sensitive strains of enterococci, viridan streptococci, methicillin-resistant and methicillin-sensitive *Staphylococcus aureus,* as well as against one-third to one-half of *Staphylococcus epidermidis* strains [17].

In addition to its effectiveness against a broad spectrum of micro-organisms, vancomycin is known to be stable at 4°C and 37°C, which are the two temperatures most commonly used for bioburden reduction step. Its potency remains unaffected after 6 hours of exposure at 37°C and 24 hours at 4°C [13]. One bank had validated vancomycin stability for up to 48 hours at 4°C. 73.3% of the banks conducted bioburden reduction in the cold (1-10°C), with the majority incubating at 4°C for 18-24 hours. Only 13.3% of the banks performed bioburden reduction step at room temperature (21°C) and the other 13.3% conducted this step at physiological temperatures (33-38°C). Regardless of the antibiotic combinations or incubation conditions used, in each case, the procedure had been validated to meet the banks' final product requirements. For these reasons, many banks are hesitant to change their protocols, especially as procedural changes would require additional validation, which can be both costly and time-consuming.

Although the current antibiotic regimens utilised by international heart valve banks is referred to as 'low dose', the concentrations of antibiotics used exceeds the minimum inhibitory concentration (MIC) of most micro-organisms [4,19]. For instance, the MIC of vancomycin is approximately 0.5-16 µg/mL against *Staphylococcus aureus* [6,17,20], 4 µg/mL against Group B streptococci (*Streptococcus agalactiae*) [17], 1 µg/mL against *Enterococcus facecalis* [6], and 0.25 µg/mL against *Bacillus subtilis* [20]. From the survey, it was revealed that 76.9% of the banks decontaminated homografts with 50 µg/mL vancomycin and 23.1% used 500 µg/mL, both of which significantly exceeds the MIC of these susceptible pathogens.

Benefits and Concerns of Residual Antibiotics

It is known that antibiotic-decontaminated homografts show increased resistance to infection [21]. There are diverse opinions as to the actual cause of this phenomenon. However, the most widely accepted view is that residual antibiotics present in the implanted homograft act prophylactically in the recipient [3,4,19]. This is particularly important when homograft replacement is used as a treatment for infective endocarditis or infection of bioprosthetic or mechanical valves [19].

Despite the potential benefits, there are concerns with regards to the presence of antibiotic residues. Firstly, there are concerns that the presence of residual antibiotics may cause an allergic or hypersensitive reaction in the recipient. Skin rashes and medication-associated fever have been reported in 1-8% of patients receiving vancomycin [17]. However, given the concentration of vancomycin used in homograft decontamination is very low as compared to therapeutic dosage, the risk to recipients of vancomycin-treated homografts is probably minimal [17,19]. In addition, vancomycin only comes into temporary contact with homografts, and most of it is removed during processing and thawing. Tissue banks accredited by the American Association of Tissue Banks (AATB) practise the rinsing of homografts in two phases - (1) after incubation in antibiotics prior to storage, and (2) after thawing of homograft prior to implantation into the recipient. Studies had demonstrated that antibiotics, such as vancomycin, are diluted to a negligible level ($\leq$0.05%) after rinsing the homograft prior to implantation [19]. Routine follow-ups on 51 recipients from the authors' tissue bank had found no cases of allergic reactions as a result of residual antibiotics or vancomycin.

Another concern is that the presence of antibiotics on post-antibiotic incubation tissue and solution samples has the potential to compromise the reliability of microbiological test methods performed to validate the tissue decontamination process [4,13,22,23]. To counteract this potential bacteriostatic/ fungastatic effect (BF effect) and ensure validity of test results, the detection system employed must either (1) contain an effective neutralising agent (for instance, blood culture bottles), and/or (2) allow sufficient rinsing with a suitable rinsing solution (for instance, in membrane filtration) to effectively remove inhibitory substances.

Microbial contamination detection systems using defined nutrient broths have shown to be effective in detecting low-level contamination in tissue and solution samples collected at various stages during homograft processing. For example, the BacTec bottle system had been validated against a range of micro-organisms listed in the British Pharmacopoeia Appendix XVI E. Microbiological Control of Cellular Products [24] and it was found to be suitable for the detection of low-level microbial contamination (<10 colony-forming units) in homografts and rinse solutions in terms of specificity and sensitivity. This type of test method contains a neutralising agent that effectively eliminates the masking of microbial contamination by residual antibiotics. The disadvantage of this type of detection system is that only a limited volume (~10 ml) of sample can be tested per bottle.

It was recommended that to counteract the BF effect and ensure a valid sterility test, 50-2000ml of solution per tissue should be tested, depending on tissue size [22]. To achieve this, the membrane filtration method is capable of testing a larger volume of solution. The filter disc can also be placed onto nutrient plates to quantitate microbial contamination levels on the tissue if required. For these reasons, membrane filtration is considered by many banks to be the gold standard for microbiological assessment of solutions [1]. In this method, an appropriate amount of test solution (10% or more of the total volume) is flushed through a size exclusion membrane capable of retaining micro-organisms. It is then transferred into a nutrient broth or placed onto a nutrient plate. The United States Pharmacopeia <71> guideline states that the filter disc's pore size should be no greater than 0.45-micron for effective microbial retention [25]. The benefits of this technique are (1) a large volume of solution can be tested, (2) should the solution contain substances that cause BF effect, such as antibiotics, rinsing the filter disc with a suitable rinse agent can eliminate most, if not all, of these inhibitory substances, and (3) bioburden levels can be quantitated, if required. However, there were few drawbacks to this method too. Firstly, it is more time-consuming than the blood bottle test system. Secondly, it is more expensive [1]. However, due to the importance of microbial contamination detection in ensuring the safety of clinical homografts, and the perception that filtration is a more robust test method than direct inoculation into culture broths, many tissue banks are adopting this method to detect microbiological contamination in homograft samples.

Conclusion

Evaluation of microbiological culture results is critical in tissue banking. The discard of only the culture-positive tissue or all tissues retrieved from the same donor is dependent on several factors. These include the species of micro-organism identified, the diversity of micro-organisms detected, the number of pre-processed and post-processed tissue and solution samples contaminated, and microbial contamination results of other tissues recovered from the same donor. All the banks have a list of "exclusion micro-organisms", consisting of highly virulent and/or spore-forming microbes [26], the presence of which in any test sample will result in tissue discard.

One of the most critical factors in processing soft-tissue products for implantation is utilising a bioburden reduction step that effectively eliminates microbial contamination on the homograft [26]. For cardiovascular homografts, incubation in a low-concentration antibiotics solution is now the most common bioburden reduction method used for decontamination. Given the importance of this step in ensuring product safety, it is essential that the procedure is validated and that the antibiotic cocktail used is effective against the microflora commonly isolated from homografts. As vancomycin has a broad antimicrobial spectrum of activity, especially in combination with other antibiotics such as the aminoglycosides, and is stable over a wide range of temperatures, an increasing number of heart valve banks are including vancomycin for this critical step of bioburden reduction. This would lead to an increase in the availability of safe, contaminant-free homografts for transplantation.

References

[1]   Van Kats, J. P.; Van Tricht, C.; Van Dijk, A.; Van der Schans, M.; Van den Bogaerdt A, et al (2010) Microbiological examination of donated human cardiac tissue in heart valve banking. *European Journal of Cardiothoracic Surgery*, 37: 163-169.

[2]   Fan, Y. D.; Van Hoeck, B.; Holovska, V.; Jashari, R (2012) Evaluation of decontamination process of heart valve and artery tissues in European Homograft Bank (EHB): A retrospective study of 1,055 cases. *Cell and Tissue Banking* 13(2): 297-304.

[3]   Gall, K.; Smith, S.; Willmette, C.; Wong, M.; O'Brien, M. (1995) Allograft heart valve sterilization: A six-year in-depth analysis of a twenty-five-year experience with low-dose antibiotics. *Journal of Thoracic and Cardiovascular Surgury* 110(3): 680-687.

[4]   Leeming, J. P.; Lovering, A. M.; Hunt, C. J. (2005) Residual antibiotics in allograft heart valve tissue samples following antibiotic disinfection. *Journal of Hospital Infection* 60: 231-234.

[5]   Jashari, R.; Tabaku, M.; Van Hoecb, B.; Cochéz, C.; Callant, M., et al (2007) Decontamination of heart valve and arterial allografts in the European Homograft Bank (EHB): comparison of two different antibiotic cocktails in low temperature conditions. *Cell and Tissue Banking* 8(4): 247-255.

[6]   Villalba, R.; Solis, F.; Fornes, G.; Jimenez A Eisman, M., et al. (2012) In vitro susceptibility of high virulence microorganisms isolated in heart valve banking. *Cell and Tissue Banking* 13: 441-445.

[7]   CDC (2003) Invasive *Streptococcus pyogenes* after allograft implantation --- Colorado, 2003. *MMWR* 52(48): 1173-1176.

[8]   Pirnay, J. P.; Verween, G.; Pascual, B.; Verbeken, G.; De Corte, P., et al (2012) Evaluation of a microbiological screening and acceptance procedure for cryopreserved skin allografts based on 14 days cultures. *Cell and Tissue Banking* 13: 287-295.

[9]   Barratt-Boyes, B. G. (1987) 25 year's clinical experience of allograft surgery – a time for reflection 1962-1987. In: Yankah AC, Hetzer R, Miller DC, Ross DN, Somerville J, Yacoub MH (eds) Cardiac valve allografts. *Springer,* New York, pp. 347-358.

[10] Tabaku, M.; Jashari, R.; Carton, H. F.; Du Verger, A.; Van Hoeck, B. et al. (2004) Processing of cardiovascular allografts: effectiveness of European Homograft Bank (EHB) antimicrobial treatment (cool

decontamination protocol with low concentration of antibiotics). *Cell and Tissue Banking* 5: 261-266.

[11] Jashari, R.; Van Hoeck, B.; Tabaku, M.; Vanderkelen, A. (2004) Banking of the human heart valves and the arteries at the European homograft bank (EHB) – overview of a 14-year activity in this International Association in Brussels. *Cell and Tissue Banking* 5: 239-251.

[12] Brockbank, K. G. M.; Siler, D. J. B. (2001) Aseptic and antiseptic treatment of donated and living engineered organs and tissues. In: Seymour SB, editor. Disinfection, Sterilization, and Preservation, 5th edition. *Lippincott Williams & Wilkins* 2001. pp. 1011-1022.

[13] Heng, W. L.; Lim, C. H.; Tan, B. H. Chlebicki, M. P.; Lee, W. H. L. et al. (2012) From penicillin-streptomycin to amikacin-vancomycin: antibiotic decontamination of cardiovascular homografts in Singapore. *PLoS ONE* 7(12): e51605. doi:10.1371/journal.pone.0051605.

[14] Germain, M.; Thibault, L.; Jacques, A.; Trembley, J.; Bourgeois, R. (2010) Heart valve allograft decontamination with antibiotics: impact of the temperature of incubation on efficacy. *Cell and Tissue Banking* 11: 197-204.

[15] Heng, W. L.; Albrecht, H.; Chiappini, P.; Lim, Y. P.; Manning, L. (2013) International heart valve bank survey: review of processing practices and activity outcomes. *Journal of Transplantation* vol. 2013, article ID 163150, 11 pages. doi:10.1155/2013/163150.

[16] Watanakunakorn, C. (1984) Mode of action and in-vitro activity of vancomycin. *Journal of Antimicrobial Chemotherapy* 14 (suppl D): 7-18.

[17] Devaro, R. E.; Glew, R. H. (2004) Vancomycin and Teicoplanin. In: Gorbach SL, Bartlett JG, Blacklow NR, editors. Infectious diseases. *Lippincott Williams & Wilkins* 2004. pp 233-241.

[18] Gilbert, D. N. (1999) Aminoglycosides. In: Root RK, editor. Clinical infectious diseases – a practical approach. *Oxford University Press Inc* 1999. pp. 273-284.

[19] Jashari, R.; Faucon, F.; Hoeck, B. V.; Gelas, S. D.; Fan, Y. (2011) Determination of residual antibiotics in cryopreserved heart valve allografts. *Transfusion Medicine and Hemotherapy* 38(6):379-386.

[20] Traub, W. H.; Leonhard, B. (1995) Heat stability of the antimicrobial activity of sixty-two antibacterial agents. *Journal of Antimicrobial Chemotherapy* 35: 149-154.

[21] Da Costa, M. L.; Ghofaili, F. A.; El Oakley, R. M. (2006) Allograft tissue for use in valve replacement. *Cell and Tissue Banking* 7: 337-348.

[22] Alexander, K.; Bryans, T. (2006) Evaluation of the sterility test for detection of microbial contaminants of allografts. *Cell and Tissue Banking* 7: 23-28.

[23] Eastlund, T. (2006) Bacterial infection transmitted by human tissue allograft transplantation. *Cell and Tissue Banking* 7(3):147-66.

[24] British Pharmacopeia Online (2012) Appendix XVI E. *Microbiological Control of Cellular Products.*

[25] United States Pharmacopeia Online (2012) <71> Sterility Tests.

[26] Ireland, L.; Spelman, D. (2005) Bacterial contamination of tissue allografts – experiences of the donor tissue bank of Victoria. *Cell and Tissue Banking* 6: 181-189.

In: Vancomycin
Editor: Abu Gafar Hossion

ISBN: 978-1-62948-559-1
© 2013 Nova Science Publishers, Inc.

Chapter 5

Common and Uncommon Adverse Effects of Vancomycin

Florent Valour[1,2], Judith Karsenty[1,3], Sandrine Leroy[1],
Anissa Bouaziz[1,3], Sarah Milley[1], Benoit Bensaid[4],
Frédéric Laurent[2,3,5], Florence Ader[1,2,3,4],
Christian Chidiac[1,2,3] and Tristan Ferry[1,2,3,],*
[1]Infectious Diseases Department, Croix-Rousse Hospital,
Hospices Civils de Lyon, France
[2]Centre International de Recherche en Infectiologie, CIRI, Lyon, France
[3]Claude Bernard University, Lyon, France
[4]Allergo-Immunology and Dermatology Department,
Hospices Civils de Lyon, France
[5]French Reference Center for Staphylococci,
Hospices Civils de Lyon, France

Abstract

The present article describes the common and uncommon adverse
effects of vancomycin. Vancomycin is reputed to be associated with a
high rate of adverse events, mainly because most tolerance studies were

* Corresponding author: Tristan Ferry – Infectious Diseases Department, 103 Grande-Rue de la
Croix-Rousse, 69004 Lyon, France. E-mail: tristan.ferry@univ-lyon1.fr.

conducted using early preparations that contained impurities. It is known to be venotoxic, and is frequently associated with thrombosis, especially if administered through a peripheral catheter. When it is administered through a central venous catheter, thrombosis is more uncommon, but may occur in association with superior vena cava syndrome. Infusion-related reactions due to histamine release when perfusion duration is less than 1 hour (red-man or red-neck syndrome) are the most frequent side effect, reported in up to 11% of patients. In recent studies, vancomycin-associated nephrotoxicity was reported in approximately 5% of patients, and was associated with high plasma levels (> 15 mg/L), concomitant use of nephrotoxic agents, long treatment durations, and possibly with intermittent infusion. The role of vancomycin in ototoxicity remains controversial, but reversible hearing loss may occur in 12% of patients, mainly in the elderly. Other vancomycin-induced adverse events include allergic reactions (2-3%), neutropenia (1-2%) and thrombocytopenia. In addition to targeting efficient plasma rates, measurement of trough plasma concentration may reduce the incidence of vancomycin-related side effects.

Keywords: Vancomycin, adverse events

Introduction

Vancomycin is usually reputed to be associated with a high toxicity rate, mainly because most tolerance studies were conducted with early preparations, which were only about 70% pure. These impurities are supposed to have contributed to a high incidence of adverse events, and especially vancomycin-related nephrotoxicity and hearing loss. A decrease in reported serious adverse events has been observed concomitantly with improvement in manufacturing processes, leading to a global incidence of vancomycin-adverse reactions near to 25% in more recent studies [1, 2].

Vancomycin-related Nephrotoxicity

Mechanism

Elimination of vancomycin is almost exclusively renal, principally via glomerular filtration, but also via active tubular secretion [3]. Some animal studies have suggested that vancomycin accumulation in proximal renal tubular cells may induce oxidative stress and mitochondrial damage, leading to cell necrosis and kidney injury, linked with acute tubulointerstitial nephritis [4, 5]. In the same mice model, changes in gene expression in the inflammation and complement pathways in response to high-dose vancomycin therapy suggested a link between vancomycin-related nephrotoxicity and complement activation [5].

Incidence

Nephrotoxicity has been associated with vancomycin since its introduction in the early 1950s, with incidence ranging from < 1% to > 40% in various studies [6, 7]. This variability is due to differences in vancomycin preparation and the level of impurities, the baseline characteristics of the study population, and dosing regimens. However, with standard doses (i.e., daily dose < 4 g or < 30 mg/kg), the incidence of nephrotoxicity seems to range from 0 to 10% [8]. Concomitant use of other nephrotoxic agents increases rates of vancomycin-associated toxicity up to as much as 35% [9, 10].

Acute Renal Failure Characteristics

Onset of acute renal failure ranges from 4 to 8 days after initiation of vancomycin [9, 11]. Mean increase in plasmatic creatinine levels ranges from 75 to 125 micromol/L, corresponding to a decrease in creatinine clearance of 35-45% [9, 12, 13]. Serum creatinine levels return to baseline in more than 70% of patients after termination of vancomycin [12,14].

Risk Factors

Risk factors for vancomycin nephrotoxicity include high doses and trough plasma concentrations, long treatment duration, multiple comorbidities, intensive care, the use of concomitant nephrotoxins, and obesity [8, 15].

Vancomycin exposure, monitored by pharmacodynamic parameters and treatment duration, is an important risk factor for nephrotoxicity. Vancomycin trough plasma level has been reported to be the most accurate pharmacodynamic indicator of nephrotoxicity risk [11]: a level of > 15 mg/L was identified as a predictor of acute kidney injury in many studies, with risk between 21% and 65% [9, 11, 12, 14, 16, 17]. However, all these studies included patients with other concomitant risk factors for renal failure, including concomitant use of other nephrotoxins. Moreover, the temporal relationship between elevated trough plasma level and onset of renal failure was not specified in most studies, leading to an unclear cause-effect relationship [18]. In addition to plasma concentration, treatment duration was reported to be a risk factor in many studies [14, 17]: beyond 14 days' treatment, the odds ratio for nephrotoxicity was 2.6 [12], with nephrotoxicity incidence increasing with the time spent with trough serum concentrations between 15 and 20 mg/L (from 6% for ≤ 7 days to 30% for > 14 days) [17].

Concomitant use of other nephrotoxins is associated with increased risk of renal toxicity, particularly in the case of aminoglycosides [16, 17, 19, 20].

Patients in intensive care have a higher risk of vancomycin-induced nephrotoxicity, especially if they have numerous comorbidities (on the APACHE II score) or receive vasopressor therapy [9, 11, 12, 21].

Obesity appears to be an independent risk factor for vancomycin-induced nephrotoxicity. Little is known about the use of antimicrobials, and especially vancomycin, in obese patients, in whom drug pharmacokinetics may vary greatly due to differences in tissue distribution, protein binding, metabolism, and clearance of antimicrobials [22]. Initial dosage should be calculated as a function of total bodyweight, but dose adjustments in obese patients may benefit from frequent monitoring of plasma drug concentrations [11, 23].

Finally, the beneficial effects of continuous infusion are controversial [24-26]. However, a recent meta-analysis, including one randomized clinical trial and five observational studies, reported a significantly lower risk of nephrotoxicity in patients with continuous then intermittent infusion, with a relative risk of 0.63 [27].

Vancomycin-related Skin Reactions

Vancomycin induces different types of hypersensitivity reaction, ranging from localized skin reactions to anaphylactic shock.

Red-man Syndrome

Red-man (or red-neck) syndrome is not a true allergic reaction, but rather a non-specific infusion-rate-dependent release of histamine linked with direct mast cell activation by vancomycin [28, 29]. Incidence varies between 3% and 13% of infected patients receiving vancomycin, but has been reported to be higher in under-40 year-olds, especially children, and in healthy volunteers [29-34]. It manifests as flushing, erythema and pruritus of the upper body (i.e., face, neck and upper torso). Severe forms may include pain and muscle spasm, dyspnea, hypotension, angioedema and paresthesia around the mouth [35, 36]. Onset is mainly in the first 10 minutes after initiation of infusion, or soon after completion, even with the first vancomycin administration. It is often associated with rapid high-dose infusion (> 500 mg over < 30 min) [32, 37], and has also been reported after oral administration of vancomycin [38]. Risk is increased with concomitant use of other agents potentiating mast cell degranulation: especially opioids, muscle relaxants, contrast dye, and other antimicrobials such as ciprofloxacin, rifampin, and amphotericin B [39, 40]. Optimal management has never been determined by randomized studies. Interruption of infusion and antihistamines are sufficient for mild reactions; infusion can then be restarted at half the original rate. Antihistamines should be given, for 4 or more hours, before future doses in patients with severe reaction, keeping in mind the difficulty of distinguishing severe red-man syndrome from real anaphylaxis. Prevention includes using a slow infusion rate (< 10 mg/min), with empiric antihistamine premedication if more rapid infusion is required or in case of previous reaction [32, 41].

IgE-mediated Anaphylaxis

Real allergic reaction involving drug-specific IgE is thought to be rare. Symptoms generally occur after repeated prior exposure and are non-specific, including urticaria, angioedema, generalized pruritus, hypotension and tachycardia, vomiting, and bronchospasm [42-44]. Plasma histamine or serum tryptase levels are poorly contributive to diagnosis as they do not discriminate between anaphylaxis and non-specific mast cell activation [32, 45]. Vancomycin skin testing has not been validated. Treatment of such allergic reactions consists in the usual management of anaphylaxis, including termination of vancomycin infusion, antihistamines, and standard resuscitation care for severe forms (epinephrine/adrenalin, intravenous fluids). Other antibiotics should be considered for patients with vancomycin-induced severe anaphylactic reaction.

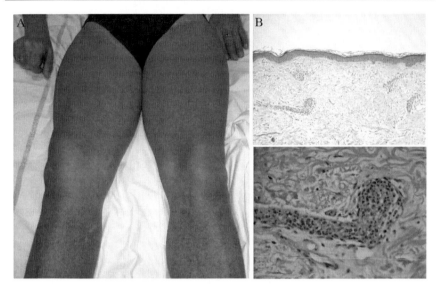

Figure 1. Skin rash during vancomycin-induced hypersensitivity syndrome (panel A), corresponding to perivascular eosinophilic infiltration on skin biopsy (panels B and C).

Drug Rash Eosinophilia with Systemic Symptoms (DRESS) or Drug-induced Hypersensitivity Syndrome (DiHS)

The incidence of DRESS syndrome has never been evaluated but it seems to occur in 1 of 1,000 to 10,000 exposures to "high-risk" drugs such as antiepileptics, with a mortality rate up to 10%. To date, only 8 cases of vancomycin-related DRESS syndrome have been reported, none of which were fatal [46, 47]. Cumulative vancomycin dose and exceedingly high serum trough levels do not seem to be related to onset of DRESS syndrome but may prolong evolution, although this remains controversial. Clinical presentation of vancomycin-induced DRESS syndrome has no specificity. Onset is after 2 to 8 weeks' exposure, and associates skin rash (figure 1) with fever, lymphadenopathy, eosinophilia, and systemic involvement such as hepatitis, nephritis and interstitial lung disease. Eosinophilia seems to be moderate with vancomycin, at 1,000 to 1,500/mm^3, whereas levels of up to 20,000/mm^3 have been reported with other treatments. Skin biopsy histology is non-specific, showing dermal perivascular lymphocytic and eosinophilic infiltration that is much denser than in other allergic skin reactions, but very variable (figure 1). Dermal edema and diffuse keratinocyte necrosis can be observed. Treatment is non-specific. Withdrawal of vancomycin is mandatory. In case of severe visceral involvement, the use of corticosteroids is empiric, with an initial dosage of between 0.5 and 1 mg/kg/day, followed by progressive decrease over several weeks.

Other Forms of Vancomycin Skin Hypersensitivity

Maculopapular or urticarial skin rash is the most common manifestation of vancomycin allergic reaction, occurring in 6 to 9% of patients [20, 48, 49, 50].

Linear IgA bullous dermatosis is a rare autoimmune vancomycin-induced adverse event, occurring from 1 day to 1 month after vancomycin administration (figure 2) [51, 52, 53]. The absence of mucosal membrane involvement usually allows it to be distinguished from toxic epidermal necrolysis [53], but direct immunofluorescence is usually needed to confirm diagnosis. All published cases showed resolution of symptoms after termination of vancomycin. Prednisone and dapsone have been proposed when no alternative treatment is available [51].

Other cutaneous reactions are rare but can be severe, including Stevens-Johnson syndrome, toxic epidermal necrolysis, exfoliative dermatitis, leukocytoclastic vasculitis, and extensive fixed drug eruption [54-59].

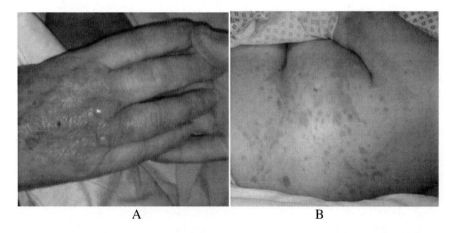

A   B

Figure 2. Vancomycin-induced linear IgA bullous dermatosis (Panels A and B).

Vancomycin Desensitization

Desensitization can be proposed in case of severe red-man syndrome or mild anaphylactic reaction, when no alternative treatment is available. This procedure is contraindicated in case of past exfoliative skin reaction or DRESS, and is generally not performed in patients with history of drug fever, hematologic or renal allergic reactions or linear IgA bullous dermatosis. A variety of desensitization protocols have been described, and must be run following the advice of an allergy specialist [30, 39, 60]. As they induce a temporary state of tolerance, they must be performed just before reintroducing vancomycin.

Vancomycin-related Ototoxicity

Ototoxicity was one of the first recorded adverse events following the beginning of clinical use of vancomycin [61]. However, vancomycin's implication in hearing loss remains controversial for several reasons: i) these first observations were associated with very high doses of vancomycin despite renal insufficiency, leading to plasma levels as high as 100 µg/mL; ii) vancomycin was not associated with ototoxicity in many animal models [62, 63]; iii) ototoxicity, like nephrotoxicity, showed a much lower incidence in the years following the introduction of purified preparations, leading some authors to consider impurities as responsible for vancomycin-associated hearing loss [63]; iv) a correlation between plasma vancomycin levels and ototoxicity, although suggested, remains unclear [8, 64-66]; and v) a final confusing factor is the frequent concomitant use of aminoglycosides, known to be highly ototoxic. For instance, Cantu et al. reviewed 53 published cases of supposed vancomycin-induced ototoxicity and concluded that vancomycin was rare implicated as a single agent [65]. Nevertheless, the frequency of vancomycin-induced ototoxicity has been reported to range from 1% to 12%, and seems to be more frequent in the elderly [64-67]. In the largest existing cohort study, the ototoxicity rate was assessed at 3% overall, reaching 6% in patients receiving other ototoxic agents [64]. The mechanism leading to vancomycin-induced hearing loss is thought to be linked to irreversible auditory nerve damage [64]. In most observed cases, however, the hearing loss was reversible within three weeks after termination of vancomycin. Vertigo and tinnitus are also occasionally reported during vancomycin therapy, and may precede hearing loss.

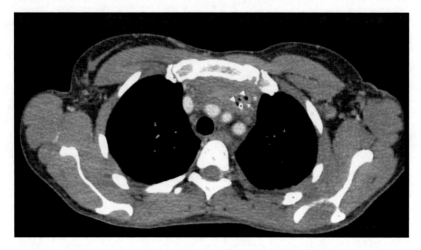

Figure 3. Computed tomography showing an aseptic central catheter (asterisk) thrombophlebitis (arrow) with gas bubbles (arrow heads) following prolonged vancomycin administration.

OTHER ADVERSE EFFECTS

Venous Toxicity

Vancomycin is known to be venotoxic. Local venous inflammation, related to low pH in the vancomycin preparation, is one of the most frequent adverse events, observed in 3 to 30% of patients [48,68]. Venotoxicity incidence seems to be reduced by increasing drug dilution and infusion period. Thrombophlebitis is a very common problem when vancomycin is administered through a peripheral venous cannula [10]. In earlier studies, thrombosis occurred in 28% of cases [69], but after the 1980s improved purification techniques decreased the rate to approximately 13% [70]. No difference was shown between continuous versus twice-daily administration [71].

Thrombophlebitis of the central catheter is possible, but occurs less frequently (in almost 3% of cases) [72]. Some cases of aseptic thrombophlebitis with gas bubbles on the central venous catheter have been reported (figure 3) [73]. These cases could be severe, with superior vena cava thrombosis that could require surgery. In comparison with twice-daily administration, continuous administration of vancomycin through a central venous catheter is suspected of inducing higher risk of aseptic thrombophlebitis, but this association has not been demonstrated. Finally, coadministration of vancomycin with penicillins is chemically incompatible (crystal formation) and may result in clogging the catheter. The catheter must be flushed after use of vancomycin, if penicillin is used.

Hematologic Disorders

Hematologic reactions caused by vancomycin include leukocytosis, eosinophilia, immune thrombocytopenia, and neutropenia. The incidence of thrombocytopenia ($< 150,000/mm^3$) has been reported to about 5-12% [74, 75, 76]. Vancomycin-induced neutropenia has also been described, with an incidence of 2% to 8%. Agranulocytosis seems to be rare, but was reported with an incidence of 3.5% in a retrospective study of outpatients receiving parenteral vancomycin therapy [74]. The interval from vancomycin initiation to onset of neutropenia ranges from 9 to 30 days. Risk does not seem to be related to serum drug concentrations but tends to increase with longer vancomycin courses, so that leukocyte count monitoring is recommended in patients receiving vancomycin for more than 2 weeks [77-83]. Vancomycin-induced thrombocytopenia and neutropenia are thought to be mainly immunologically mediated. Rapid and complete recovery usually ensues once vancomycin administration is discontinued.

Hepatic Reactions

The absence of significant hepatic metabolism of vancomycin probably explains why vancomycin is associated with only minor transient asymptomatic elevation of plasma aminotransferase levels in about 1% to 9% of patients. Most hepatic reactions are in fact associated with more severe systemic reaction such as DRESS or Stevens Johnson syndrome [84].

Drug-induced Fever

Finally, vancomycin can be responsible for drug-induced fever in 2% of cases [70, 82, 85].

Conclusion

In conclusion, despite the acceptable impurity rate of present-day vancomycin preparations, clinical use of vancomycin is still associated with a high incidence of side effects, occurring in nearly a quarter of patients. The most common of them, however, including infusion-related reactions, are generally benign and can be prevented. Renal failure occurs in less than 10% of patients, and appears to be reversible in most cases. Close monitoring of vancomycin trough concentration may help to control the risk of vancomycin-induced kidney injury, especially in at-risk patients. The implication of vancomycin in hearing loss remains uncertain, but clinicians should be vigilant, especially when vancomycin is used in association with other ototoxic agents such as aminoglycosides. Finally, particular attention should be paid to the underestimated risk of vancomycin-associated hematologic disorders and thrombosis.

Acknowledgments

(On behalf of the Lyon Bone and Joint Infection Study Group)

We acknowledge our colleagues in the Lyon Bone and Joint Infection Study Group: *Physicians* – Tristan Ferry, Thomas Perpoint, André Boibieux, François Biron, Florence Ader, Anissa Bouaziz, Judith Karsenty, Fatiha Daoud, Johanna Lippman, Evelyne Braun, Marie-Paule Vallat, Patrick Miailhes, Florent Valour, Christian Chidiac, Dominique Peyramond; *Surgeons* – Sébastien Lustig, Franck Trouillet, Philippe Neyret, Olivier Guyen, Gualter Vaz, Christophe Lienhart, Michel-Henry Fessy, Cédric Barrey; *Microbiologists* – Frédéric Laurent, François Vandenesch, Jean-Philippe Rasigade; *Nuclear Medicine* – Isabelle Morelec, Emmanuel Deshayes, Marc Janier, Francesco Giammarile; *PK/PD specialists* – Michel Tod, Marie-Claude Gagnieu, Sylvain Goutelle; *Clinical Research Assistant* – Eugénie Mabrut.

REFERENCES

[1]   Marinho, D. S.; Huf, G.; Ferreira, B. L.; Castro, H.; Rodrigues, C. R.; de Sousa, V. P. et al. The study of vancomycin use and its adverse reactions

associated to patients of a Brazilian university hospital. *BMC Res. Notes* 2011;4:236.

[2]   Wood, M. J. The comparative efficacy and safety of teicoplanin and vancomycin. *J. Antimicrob. Chemother.* 1996;37:209-22.

[3]   Nakamura, T.; Takano, M.; Yasuhara, M.; Inui, K. In-vivo clearance study of vancomycin in rats. *J. Pharm. Pharmacol.* 1996;48:1197-200.

[4]   Oktem, F.; Arslan, M. K.; Ozguner, F.; Candir, O.; Yilmaz, H. R.; Ciris, M. et al. In vivo evidences suggesting the role of oxidative stress in pathogenesis of vancomycin-induced nephrotoxicity: protection by erdosteine. *Toxicology* 2005;215:227-33.

[5]   Dieterich, C.; Puey, A,; Lin, S.; Swezey, R.; Furimsky, A.; Fairchild, D. et al. Gene expression analysis reveals new possible mechanisms of vancomycin-induced nephrotoxicity and identifies gene markers candidates. *Toxicol. Sci.* 2009;107:258-69.

[6]   Gupta, A.; Biyani, M.; Khaira, A. Vancomycin nephrotoxicity: myths and facts. *Neth. J. Med.* 2011;69:379-83.

[7]   Hazlewood, K. A.; Brouse, S. D.; Pitcher, W. D.; Hall, R. G. Vancomycin-associated nephrotoxicity: grave concern or death by character assassination? *Am. J. Med.* 2010;123:182 e1-7.

[8]   Rybak, M.; Lomaestro, B.; Rotschafer, J. C.; Moellering, R. Jr.; Craig, W.; Billeter, M. et al. Therapeutic monitoring of vancomycin in adult patients: a consensus review of the American Society of Health-System Pharmacists, the Infectious Diseases Society of America, and the Society of Infectious Diseases Pharmacists. *Am. J. Health Syst. Pharm.* 2009;66:82-98.

[9]   Lodise, T. P.; Lomaestro, B.; Graves, J.; Drusano, G. L. Larger vancomycin doses (at least four grams per day) are associated with an increased incidence of nephrotoxicity. *Antimicrob. Agents Chemother.* 2008;52:1330-6.

[10]   Sorrell, T. C.; Collignon, P. J. A prospective study of adverse reactions associated with vancomycin therapy. *J. Antimicrob. Chemother.* 1985;16:235-41.

[11]   Lodise, T. P.; Patel, N.; Lomaestro, B. M.; Rodvold, K. A.; Drusano, G. L. Relationship between initial vancomycin concentration-time profile and nephrotoxicity among hospitalized patients. *Clin Infect Dis* 2009;49:507-14.

[12]   Jeffres, M. N.; Isakow, W.; Doherty, J. A.; Micek, S. T.; Kollef, M. H. A retrospective analysis of possible renal toxicity associated with

vancomycin in patients with health care-associated methicillin-resistant Staphylococcus aureus pneumonia. *Clin. Ther.* 2007;29:1107-15.

[13] Kralovicova, K; Spanik, S.; Halko, J.; Netriova, J.; Studena-Mrazova, M.; Novotny, J. et al. Do vancomycin serum levels predict failures of vancomycin therapy or nephrotoxicity in cancer patients? *J. Chemother.* 1997;9:420-6.

[14] Pritchard, L.; Baker, C.; Leggett, J.; Sehdev, P.; Brown, A.; Bayley, K. B. Increasing vancomycin serum trough concentrations and incidence of nephrotoxicity. *Am. J. Med.* 2010;123:1143-9.

[15] Elyasi, S.; Khalili, H.; Dashti-Khavidaki, S.; Mohammadpour, A. Vancomycin-induced nephrotoxicity: mechanism, incidence, risk factors and special populations. A literature review. *Eur. J. Clin. Pharmacol.* 2012;68:1243-55.

[16] Hermsen, E. D.; Hanson, M.; Sankaranarayanan, J.; Stoner, J. A.; Florescu, M. C.; Rupp, M. E. Clinical outcomes and nephrotoxicity associated with vancomycin trough concentrations during treatment of deep-seated infections. *Expert Opin. Drug Saf.* 2010;9:9-14.

[17] Hidayat, L. K.; Hsu, D. I.; Quist, R.; Shriner, K. A.; Wong-Beringer, A. High-dose vancomycin therapy for methicillin-resistant Staphylococcus aureus infections: efficacy and toxicity. *Arch. Intern. Med.* 2006;166:2138-44.

[18] Rybak, M. J.; Lomaestro, B. M.; Rotschafer, J. C.; Moellering, R. C.; Craig, W. A.; Billeter, M. et al. Vancomycin therapeutic guidelines: a summary of consensus recommendations from the infectious diseases Society of America, the American Society of Health-System Pharmacists, and the Society of Infectious Diseases Pharmacists. *Clin. Infect. Dis.* 2009;49:325-7.

[19] Rybak, M. J.; Albrecht, L. M.; Boike, S. C.; Chandrasekar, P. H. Nephrotoxicity of vancomycin, alone and with an aminoglycoside. *J. Antimicrob. Chemother.* 1990;25:679-87.

[20] Wood, C. A.; Kohlhepp, S. J.; Kohnen, P. W.; Houghton, D. C.; Gilbert, D. N. Vancomycin enhancement of experimental tobramycin nephrotoxicity. *Antimicrob. Agents Chemother.* 1986;30:20-4.

[21] McKamy, S.; Hernandez, E.; Jahng, M.; Moriwaki, T.; Deveikis, A.; Le, J. Incidence and risk factors influencing the development of vancomycin nephrotoxicity in children. *J. Pediatr.* 2011;158:422-6.

[22] Pai, M. P.; Bearden, D. T. Antimicrobial dosing considerations in obese adult patients. *Pharmacotherapy* 2007;27:1081-91.

[23]　Falagas, M. E.; Karageorgopoulos, D. E. Adjustment of dosing of antimicrobial agents for bodyweight in adults. *Lancet* 2010;375:248-51

[24]　Hutschala, D.; Kinstner, C.; Skhirdladze, K.; Thalhammer, F.; Muller, M.; Tschernko, E. Influence of vancomycin on renal function in critically ill patients after cardiac surgery: continuous versus intermittent infusion. *Anesthesiology* 2009;111:356-65.

[25]　Ingram, P. R.; Lye, D. C.; Fisher, D. A.; Goh, W. P.; Tam, V. H. Nephrotoxicity of continuous versus intermittent infusion of vancomycin in outpatient parenteral antimicrobial therapy. *Int. J. Antimicrob. Agents* 2009;34:570-4.

[26]　Vuagnat, A.; Stern, R.; Lotthe, A.; Schuhmacher, H.; Duong, M.; Hoffmeyer, P. et al. High dose vancomycin for osteomyelitis: continuous vs. intermittent infusion. *J. Clin. Pharm. Ther.* 2004;29:351-7.

[27]　Cataldo, M. A.; Tacconelli, E.; Grilli, E.; Pea, F.; Petrosillo, N. Continuous versus intermittent infusion of vancomycin for the treatment of Gram-positive infections: systematic review and meta-analysis. *J. Antimicrob. Chemother.* 2012;67:17-24

[28]　Horinouchi, Y.; Abe, K.; Kubo, K.; Oka, M. Mechanisms of vancomycin-induced histamine release from rat peritoneal mast cells. *Agents Actions* 1993;40:28-36.

[29]　Wallace, M. R.; Mascola, J. R.; Oldfield, E. C. 3rd. Red man syndrome: incidence, etiology, and prophylaxis. *J. Infect. Dis.* 1991;164:1180-5.

[30]　Wazny, L. D.; Daghigh, B. Desensitization protocols for vancomycin hypersensitivity. *Ann. Pharmacother.* 2001;35:1458-64.

[31]　Korman, T. M.; Turnidge, J. D.; Grayson, M. L. Risk factors for adverse cutaneous reactions associated with intravenous vancomycin. *J. Antimicrob. Chemother.* 1997;39:371-81.

[32]　Polk, R. E.; Healy, D. P.; Schwartz, L. B.; Rock, D. T.; Garson, M. L.; Roller, K. Vancomycin and the red-man syndrome: pharmacodynamics of histamine release. *J. Infect. Dis.* 1988;157:502-7.

[33]　Wallace, M. R.; Oldfield, E. C. 3rd. Prospective evaluation of red man syndrome. *J Infect Dis* 1994;169:700-1.

[34]　O'Sullivan, T. L.; Ruffing, M. J.; Lamp, K. C.; Warbasse, L. H.; Rybak, M. J. Prospective evaluation of red man syndrome in patients receiving vancomycin. *J. Infect. Dis.* 1993;168:773-6.

[35]　Hepner, D. L.; Castells, M. C. Anaphylaxis during the perioperative period. *Anesth. Analg.* 2003;97:1381-95.

[36]   Symons, N. L.; Hobbes, A. F.; Leaver, H. K. Anaphylactoid reactions to vancomycin during anaesthesia: two clinical reports. *Can. Anaesth. Soc. J.* 1985;32:178-81.

[37]   Healy, D. P.; Sahai, J. V.; Fuller, S. H.; Polk, R. E. Vancomycin-induced histamine release and "red man syndrome": comparison of 1- and 2-hour infusions. *Antimicrob. Agents Chemother.* 1990;34:550-4.

[38]   Bergeron, L.; Boucher, F. D. Possible red-man syndrome associated with systemic absorption of oral vancomycin in a child with normal renal function. *Ann. Pharmacother.* 1994;28:581-4.

[39]   Wong, J. T.; Ripple, R. E.; MacLean, J. A.; Marks, D. R.; Bloch, K. J. Vancomycin hypersensitivity: synergism with narcotics and "desensitization" by a rapid continuous intravenous protocol. *J. Allergy Clin. Immunol.* 1994;94:189-94.

[40]   Wilson, A. P. Comparative safety of teicoplanin and vancomycin. *Int. J. Antimicrob. Agents* 1998;10:143-52.

[41]   Renz, C. L.; Thurn, J. D.; Finn, H. A.; Lynch, J. P.; Moss, J. Antihistamine prophylaxis permits rapid vancomycin infusion. *Crit. Care Med* 1999;27:1732-7.

[42]   Anne, S.; Middleton, E. Jr.; Reisman, R. E. Vancomycin anaphylaxis and successful desensitization. *Ann. Allergy* 1994;73:402-4.

[43]   Hassaballa, H.; Mallick, N.; Orlowski, J. Vancomycin anaphylaxis in a patient with vancomycin-induced red man syndrome. *Am. J. Ther.* 2000;7:319-20.

[44]   Chopra, N.; Oppenheimer, J.; Derimanov, G. S.; Fine, P. L. Vancomycin anaphylaxis and successful desensitization in a patient with end stage renal disease on hemodialysis by maintaining steady antibiotic levels. *Ann. Allergy Asthma Immunol.* 2000;84:633-5.

[45]   Renz, C. L.; Laroche, D.; Thurn, J. D.; Finn, H. A.; Lynch, J. P.; Thisted, R. et al. Tryptase levels are not increased during vancomycin-induced anaphylactoid reactions. *Anesthesiology* 1998;89:620-5.

[46]   Vauthey, L.; Uckay, I.; Abrassart, S.; Bernard, L.; Assal, M.; Ferry, T. et al. Vancomycin-induced DRESS syndrome in a female patient. *Pharmacology* 2008;82:138-41.

[47]   Diaz-Mancebo, R.; Costero-Fernandez, O.; Vega-Cabrera, C.; Olea-Tejero, T.; Yebenes, L.; Picazo, M. L. et al. Dress syndrome and acute tubulointerstitial nephritis after treatment with vancomycin and beta-lactams. Case report and literature review. *Nefrologia* 2012;32:685-7.

[48]   Finch, R. G.; Eliopoulos, G. M. Safety and efficacy of glycopeptide antibiotics. *J. Antimicrob. Chemother.* 2005;55 Suppl 2:ii5-13.

[49]   An, S. Y.; Hwang, E. K.; Kim, J. H.; Kim, J. E.; Jin, H. J.; Jin, S. M. et
       al. Vancomycin-associated spontaneous cutaneous adverse drug
       reactions. *Allergy Asthma Immunol. Res.* 2011;3:194-8.
[50]   Perrin-Lamarre, A.; Petitpain, N.; Trechot, P.; Cuny, J. F.; Schmutz, J.
       L.; Barbaud, A. Glycopeptide-induced cutaneous adverse reaction:
       results of an immunoallergic investigation in eight patients. *Ann.
       Dermatol. Venereol.* 2010;137:101-5.
[51]   Bitman, L. M.; Grossman, M. E.; Ross, H. Bullous drug eruption treated
       with amputation. A challenging case of vancomycin-induced linear IgA
       disease. *Arch. Dermatol.* 1996;132:1289-90.
[52]   Nousari, H. C.; Kimyai-Asadi, A.; Caeiro, J. P.; Anhalt, G. J. Clinical,
       demographic, and immunohistologic features of vancomycin-induced
       linear IgA bullous disease of the skin. Report of 2 cases and review of
       the literature. *Medicine (Baltimore)* 1999;78:1-8.
[53]   Coelho, S.; Tellechea, O.; Reis, J. P.; Mariano, A. Figueiredo A.
       Vancomycin-associated linear IgA bullous dermatosis mimicking toxic
       epidermal necrolysis. *Int. J. Dermatol.* 2006;45:995-6.
[54]   Laurencin, C. T.; Horan, R. F.; Senatus, P. B.; Wheeler, C. B.; Lipson,
       S. J. Stevens-Johnson-type reaction with vancomycin treatment. *Ann.
       Pharmacother.* 1992;26:1520-1.
[55]   Neal, D.; Morton, R.; Bailie, G. R.; Waldek, S. Exfoliative reaction to
       vancomycin. *Br. Med. J. (Clin. Res. Ed.)* 1988;296:137.
[56]   Alexander, II.; Greenberger, P. A. Vancomycin-induced Stevens-
       Johnson syndrome. *Allergy Asthma Proc.* 1996;17:75-8.
[57]   Vidal, C.; Gonzalez Quintela, A.; Fuente, R. Toxic epidermal necrolysis
       due to vancomycin. *Ann. Allergy* 1992;68:345-7.
[58]   Gilmore, E. S.; Friedman, J. S.; Morrell, D. S. Extensive fixed drug
       eruption secondary to vancomycin. *Pediatr. Dermatol.* 2004;21:600-2.
[59]   Felix-Getzik, E.; Sylvia, L. M. Vancomycin-induced leukocytoclastic
       vasculitis. *Pharmacotherapy* 2009;29:846-51.
[60]   Lerner, A.; Dwyer, J. M. Desensitization to vancomycin. *Ann. Intern.
       Med.* 1984;100:157.
[61]   Geraci, J. E.; Heilman, F. R.; Nichols, D. R.; Wellman, W. E. Antibiotic
       therapy of bacterial endocarditis. VII. Vancomycin for acute
       micrococcal endocarditis; preliminary report. *Proc. Staff. Meet. Mayo
       Clin.* 1958;33:172-81.
[62]   Davis, R. R.; Brummett, R. E.; Bendrick, T. W.; Himes, D. L. The
       ototoxic interaction of viomycin, capreomycin and polymyxin B with
       ethacrynic acid. *Acta Otolaryngol.* 1982;93:211-7.

[63] Tange, R. A.; Kieviet, H. L.; von Marle, J.; Bagger-Sjoback, D.; Ring, W. An experimental study of vancomycin-induced cochlear damage. *Arch. Otorhinolaryngol.* 1989;246:67-70.

[64] Bailie, G. R.; Neal, D. Vancomycin ototoxicity and nephrotoxicity. A review. *Med. Toxicol. Adverse Drug Exp.* 1988;3:376-86.

[65] Cantu, T. G. Yamanaka-Yuen NA, Lietman PS. Serum vancomycin concentrations: reappraisal of their clinical value. *Clin. Infect. Dis.* 1994;18:533-43.

[66] Forouzesh, A.; Moise, P. A. Sakoulas G. Vancomycin ototoxicity: a reevaluation in an era of increasing doses. *Antimicrob. Agents Chemother.* 2009;53:483-6.

[67] Brummett, R. E.; Fox, K. E. Vancomycin- and erythromycin-induced hearing loss in humans. *Antimicrob. Agents Chemother.* 1989;33:791-6.

[68] Wood, M. J. Comparative safety of teicoplanin and vancomycin. *J. Chemother.* 2000;12 Suppl 5:21-5.

[69] Woodley, D. W.; Hall, W. H. The treatment of severe staphylococcal infections with vancomycin. *Ann. Intern. Med.* 1961;55:235-49.

[70] Farber, B. F.; Moellering, R. C. Jr. Retrospective study of the toxicity of preparations of vancomycin from 1974 to 1981. *Antimicrob. Agents Chemother.* 1983;23:138-41.

[71] Cohen, E.; Dadashev, A.; Drucker, M.; Samra, Z.; Rubinstein, E.; Garty, M. Once-daily versus twice-daily intravenous administration of vancomycin for infections in hospitalized patients. *J Antimicrob Chemother* 2002;49:155-60.

[72] Elting, L. S.; Rubenstein, E. B.; Kurtin, D.; Rolston, K. V.; Fangtang, J.; Martin, C. G. et al. Mississippi mud in the 1990s: risks and outcomes of vancomycin-associated toxicity in general oncology practice. *Cancer* 1998;83:2597-607.

[73] Leroy, S.; Piquet, P.; Chidiac, C.; Ferry, T. Extensive thrombophlebitis with gas associated with continuous infusion of vancomycin through a central venous catheter. *BMJ Case Rep.* 2012;2012.

[74] Pai, M. P.; Mercier, R. C.; Koster, S. A. Epidemiology of vancomycin-induced neutropenia in patients receiving home intravenous infusion therapy. *Ann. Pharmacother.* 2006;40:224-8.

[75] Nasraway, S. A.; Shorr, A. F.; Kuter, D. J.; O'Grady, N.; Le, V. H.; Cammarata, S. K. Linezolid does not increase the risk of thrombocytopenia in patients with nosocomial pneumonia: comparative analysis of linezolid and vancomycin use. *Clin. Infect Dis.* 2003;37:1609-16.

[76] Rao, N.; Ziran, B. H.; Wagener, M. M.; Santa, E. R.; Yu, V. L. Similar hematologic effects of long-term linezolid and vancomycin therapy in a prospective observational study of patients with orthopedic infections. *Clin. Infect. Dis.* 2004;38:1058-64.

[77] Henry, K.; Steinberg, I.; Crossley, K. B. Vancomycin-induced neutropenia during treatment of osteomyelitis in an outpatient. *Drug Intell. Clin. Pharm.* 1986;20:783-5.

[78] Adrouny, A.; Meguerditchian, S.; Koo, C. H.; Gadallah, M.; Rasgon, S.; Idroos, M. *et al.* Agranulocytosis related to vancomycin therapy. *Am. J. Med.* 1986;81:1059-61.

[79] Koo, K. B.; Bachand, R. L.; Chow, A. W. Vancomycin-induced neutropenia. *Drug Intell. Clin. Pharm.* 1986;20:780-2.

[80] Smith, P. F.; Taylor, C. T. Vancomycin-induced neutropenia associated with fever: similarities between two immune-mediated drug reactions. *Pharmacotherapy* 1999;19:240-4.

[81] Black, E.; Lau, T. T.; Ensom, M. H. Vancomycin-induced neutropenia: is it dose- or duration-related? *Ann. Pharmacother.* 2011;45:629-38.

[82] Rocha, J. L.; Kondo, W.; Baptista, M. I.; Da Cunha, C. A.; Martins, L. T. Uncommon vancomycin-induced side effects. *Braz. J. Infect. Dis.* 2002;6:196-200.

[83] Zenon, G. J.; Cadle, R. M.; Hamill, R. J. Vancomycin-induced thrombocytopenia. *Arch. Intern. Med.* 1991;151:995-6.

[84] Chen, Y.; Yang, X. Y.; Zeckel, M.; Killian, C.; Hornbuckle, K.; Regev, A. *et al.* Risk of hepatic events in patients treated with vancomycin in clinical studies: a systematic review and meta-analysis. *Drug Saf.* 2011;34:73-82.

[85] Clayman, M. D.; Capaldo, R. A. Vancomycin allergy presenting as fever of unknown origin. *Arch. Intern. Med.* 1989;149:1425-6.

In: Vancomycin
Editor: Abu Gafar Hossion

ISBN: 978-1-62948-559-1
© 2013 Nova Science Publishers, Inc.

Chapter 6

Clinical Use of Vancomycin in Methicillin-Resistant *S. Aureus* or Coagulase-Negative Staphylococci Bacteremia, Catheter-Related Bacteremia and Endocarditis

*Alicia Marquet[1], Florent Valour[1,2], Anissa Bouaziz[1,3],
Judith Karsenty[1,3], Florence Ader[1,2,3],
Christian Chidiac[1,2,3] and Tristan Ferry[1,2,3,*]*
[1]Infectious diseases department, Croix-Rousse Hospital,
Hospices Civils de Lyon, France
[2]Centre International de Recherche en Infectiologie, CIRI, Inserm U1111,
CNRS UMR5308, ENS de Lyon, UCBL1, Lyon, France
[3]Université Claude Bernard Lyon 1, Lyon, France

* Corresponding author: Tristan Ferry – Infectious Diseases department, Croix-rousse Hospital, 103 Grande-Rue de la Croix-Rousse, 69004 Lyon, France. Email: tristan.ferry@univ-lyon1.fr.

Abstract

The clinical use of vancomycin in methicillin-resistant *S. aureus* or coagulase-negative staphylococci bacteremia, catheter-related bacteremia and endocarditis has been developed in this chapter. These methicillin-resistant *S. aureus* or coagulase-negative staphylococci bacteremia, catheter-related bacteremia and endocarditis pathogens are mainly related with health-care associated infections, and particularly catheter-related infections.

Coagulase-negative staphylococci are considered to be less virulent than *S. aureus*, as they are less frequently associated with complications and mortality. Methicillin-resistant staphylococci isolated from blood cultures are usually susceptible to vancomycin with a minimal inhibitory concentration (MIC) ≤ 2 µg/mL for *S. aureus* and ≤ 4µg/mL for coagulase-negative staphylococci. Vancomycin remained the treatment of choice of such infections.

However, as vancomycin has a slow bactericidal activity, clinicians have to adequately prescribe vancomycin, to avoid acquisition of resistance under therapy and facilitate the cure. Several reports indicate that in the range of susceptibility, high MICs (i.e between 1.5 and 2 µg/mL for *S. aureus*) are associated with a higher risk of relapse or death. Area under the curve (AUC)/MIC is the stronger predictive pharmacokinetic parameter for vancomycin efficacy in patients with bacteremia.

An AUC/MIC ratio ≥ 400 is considered to be adequate to obtain clinical effectiveness, whereas trough serum concentration at the equilibrium is the most accurate method to evaluate the vancomycin effectiveness. A trough serum of 20 mg/L allows obtaining an AUC/MIC ratio ≥ 400, even if the MIC of the isolate is close to the susceptibility breakpoint. Vancomycin has to be administered intravenously, through a central venous catheter (a peripheral access could be used during the first days of therapy), with a dosage of 15 mg/kg/d twice a day. Uncomplicated methicillin-resistant *S. aureus* or coagulase-negative staphylococci bacteremia requires at least 14 days of vancomycin therapy.

The duration of the therapy should be prolonged in uncomplicated *S. aureus* bacteremia if patients have diabetes, or receive immunosuppressive drugs. In patients with *S. aureus* catheter-related bacteremia, the catheter has always to be removed, whereas vancomycin lock therapy can be used in patients with uncomplicated methicillin-resistant coagulase-negative staphylococci catheter-related infections, in conjunction with systemic vancomycin therapy. For vancomycin lock therapy, vancomycin is combined with heparin and instilled into each catheter lumen, each day during 14 days.

In patients with complicated catheter-related bacteremia and native valve endocarditis, the duration of the vancomycin therapy has to be prolonged to 6 weeks, and has to be combined with gentamicin during 3-5 days. In patients with prosthetic valve endocarditis, vancomycin has to be combined with gentamicin during 14 days, and with rifampin during the 6 weeks.

Keywords: Staphylococci, vancomycin, bacteremia, catheter-related bacteremia, endocartidis

Introduction

S. aureus and coagulase-negative staphylococci are frequently involved in health-care associated infections, and particularly bacteremia, catheter-related bacteremia, and endocarditis. Coagulase-negative staphylococci (i.e. *S. epidermidis, S. capitis, S. warnerii*, etc.) are less virulent than *S. aureus*, as they do not produce pathogenic extracellular toxin, such as particular hemolysins and leukocidins, and are less frequently associated with severe sepsis and septic shock.

As a results, Coagulase-negative staphylococci are less frequently associated with complications and mortality, in comparison wth *S. aureus* [1, 2]. Otherwise, methicillin-resistance is associated with a worse prognosis, particularly in *S. aureus* severe infections, making their management challenging [3, 4].

The aim of this chapter was to review the clinical use of vancomycin in methicillin-resistant *S. aureus* or coagulase-negative staphylococci bacteremia, catheter-related bacteremia and endocarditis.

Methicillin-Resistant Staphylococci Primary Bacteremia

Primary bacteremia (i.e. a bacteremia not related with a catheter infection nor a postoperative infection) could be observed with all staphylococci, but *S. aureus* is the most often involved. Methicillin-resistant *S. aureus* (MRSA) primary bacteremia is mainly acquired in the hospital setting, but could also be acquired in the community, especially since particular MRSA clones, responsible for severe skin and soft tissue infection, disseminate in the community setting (MRSA clone named USA300 in the USA and MRSA clone named ST80 in Europe) [5].

Vancomycin remains the treatment of choice of methicillin-resistant staphylococci [6, 7]. However, as vancomycin has a slow bactericidal activity and a poor tissue penetration after systemic administration, clinicians have to adequately prescribe vancomycin, to avoid acquisition of resistance under therapy and facilitate the cure [8, 9]. For that purpose, it is crucial to determine the vancomycin minimal inhibitory concentration (MIC) of the responsible strain. Methicillin-resistant staphylococci isolated from blood cultures are usually susceptible to vancomycin with a minimal inhibitory concentration (MIC) ≤ 2 µg/mL for *S. aureus* and ≤ 4µg/mL for coagulase-negative staphylococci [10].

Several reports indicate that in the range of susceptibility, high MICs (i.e between 1.5 and 2 µg/mL for *S. aureus*) may be predictive of increased risk for treatment failure, longer duration of bacteremia, and thus increased risk of relapse or death [11–13]. Moreover, there is growing evidence of an evolutionary change in *S. aureus*, including the worlwide emergence of vancomycin-intermediate *S. aureus* (VISA, with MIC : 4–16 µg/mL), hetero-VISA (strains with MIC ≤ 2 µg/mL, but containing subpopulations growing at higher concentrations), and some highly vancomycin-resistant *S.aureus* (VRSA, with MIC ≥ 16 µg/mL) [14, 15]. This phenomenom, although rare, is associated with poor clinical outcomes and requires new approaches to treatment [16, 17].

Focusing on the use of vancomycin in susceptible strains, consider the pharmacokinetic parameters is crucial for the treatment of methicillin-resistant staphylococci bacteremia. Vancomycin serum concentration are routinely performed, but when to order and how to interpret the assay have been debated during decades.

Vancomycin is a concentration-independent killer, unlike aminoglycosides, and traditionnaly, vancomycin has been thought to have similar pharmacokinetic characteristics than beta-lactam antibiotics, as both target the peptidoglycans.

A varierty of pharmacokinetic and pharmacodynamic monitoring parameters has been proposed for vancomycin, including: (i) the time that the concentration of vancomycin remains above the MIC (t>MIC); (ii) the ratio of the maximum drug concentration and the MIC (C_{max}/MIC); and (iii) a combination of both t>MIC and C_{max}/MIC named area under the serum concentration-versus-time curve and the MIC (AUC/MIC). In fact, AUC/MIC is the stronger predictive pharmacokinetic parameter for vancomycin efficacy in animal models (neutropenic mouse model) and in patients with bacteremia. Indeed, two clinical studies found that an AUC/MIC ratio ≥ 400 was adequate to obtain clinical effectiveness and microbiological eradication [18-21]. In clinical practice, as it is not feasable to determine the AUC/MIC ratio, most of physicians use (i) the trough serum vancomycin concentration if vancomycin is administered intermittently (i.e a 1 hour infusion every 12h); or (ii) the 'plateau' serum vancomycin concentration if vancomycin is administered continously.

There is few data on the continuous infusion of vancomycin, and benefits and specific putative adverse events due to this way of administration have been underexplored to date. A trough or plateau serum vancomycin concentrations of at least 20 mg/L allows obtaining an AUC/MIC ratio ≥ 400, if the MIC of the isolate is < 2 µg/mL [21].

However, if an MRSA strain responsible for bacteremia has an vancomycin MIC of 2 µg/mL (breackpoint), it would be difficult to achieve the goal of AUC/MIC ratio ≥ 400, as a plateau level of 33 µg/mL is needed when the drug is administered continuously [21]. This point explains why the incidence of treatment failure is high with such isolates. As a consequence, alternative therapy to vancomycin could be more appropriate for the treatment of MRSA bacteremia, if the vancomycin MIC of the strain is 2 µg/mL. In clinical practice, trough or plateau serum concentrations at the equilibrium, as it is predictive of AUC/CMI, is the most accurate and practical method for monitoring vancomycin [21].

Monitoring of trough serum concentrations is therefore recommended for serious infections, to optimize vancomycin pharmacodynamics, improve tissue penetration, minimize selection of resistant strains, but also to reduce the risk of nephrotoxicity as part of prolonged courses of therapy, with high doses, or for patients with unstable renal function or receiving other nephrotoxic treatment [21, 22]. Monitoring of peak serum vancomycin concentration is not recommended [22].

Vancomycin has to be administered intravenously, through a central venous catheter (a peripheral access could be used fairly during the first days of therapy), with a dosage of 30 mg/kg/day including for obese patients, in two, three or four injections.

Patients receiving > 4g per day should be closely monitered, as they are at high risk of toxicity [21, 22]. Vancomycin is generally diluted in 100 to 250 mL of 5% dextrose or 0.9% saline solution with a concentration < 5mg/mL and infused at a rate not exceeding 15 mg/min, i.e 500 mg in 30 min and 1g in one hour. Because time above MIC is not the primary predictor of efficacy, continuous infusion vancomycin regimens in patients with sepsis or endocarditis are not recommended [23, 24].

A loading dose of 25 mg/kg can be administered to quickly achieve the target trough concentration in case of serious infection and to reduce the risk of emergence of VISA [21]. Prompt initiation of intravenous bactericidal therapy improves the prognosis [25].

The first trough serum concentration should be obtained just before the fourth dose, at steady-state conditions, with a target of 15–20 mg/L (6, 21, 26). In contrast to many other bacterial infections, *S. aureus* infections often require a prolonged course of treatment because of the risk of late-onset complications [6].

Uncomplicated methicillin-resistant coagulase-negative staphylococci and *S. aureus* bacteremia require at least 7 and 14 days of vancomycin therapy, respectively [28, 29, 30, 31]. Uncomplicated bacteremia is defined by the following criteria: (i) negative follow-up blood culture results (2–4 days after the initial set); (ii) defervescence within 72 h after initiation of therapy; (iii) no implanted devices (eg, prosthetic valves, cardiac or intravascular devices, and arthroplasties); (iv) no evidence of metastatic sites of infection; and (v) exclusion of endocarditis [21, 25, 32]. Transthoracic echocardiography (TTE) should be performed in all patients with *S. aureus* bacteremia, and transesophageal echocardiography (TEE) is so recommended, at least 5-7 days after onset of bacteremia, for patients who had endocarditis in the past, who have prosthetic valves, or cardiac or intravascular devices, who have clinical signs of endocarditis, who have positive follow-up blood culture results, and for all patients with MRSA bacteremia [33, 34, 35].

Methicillin-Resistant Staphylococci Catheter-Related Bacteremia

Catheter-related bacteremia is usually defined by the following criteria: (i) clinical manifestations of infection (such as fever, chills, w/o hypotension); and (ii) >1 positive blood culture results obtained from the peripheral vein and from the catheter, with a differential time to positivity (growth in a culture of blood obtained through a catheter hub is detected by an automated blood culture system at least 2 hours earlier than a culture of simultaneously drawn peripheral blood of equal volume) [36].

There is some differences in the management if the patient had MRSA vs. methicillin-resistant coagulase-negative staphylococci catheter-related bacteremia, and if the patients had complicated vs. uncomplicated (bloodstream infection and fever resolves with 72 hours in a patient who has no other intravascular hardware and no evidence of endocarditis or suppurative thrombophlebitis and no secondary hematogenous infection) catheter-related bacteremia [36].

MRSA Catheter-Related Bacteremia

In patients with MRSA catheter-related bacteremia, the catheter, whether it is a short-term central venous catheter or a long-term central venous catheter, has to be removed as quickly as possible, and the patient has to receive intravenous vancomycin therapy for at least 14 days [36].

Methicillin-Resistant Coagulase-Negative Staphylococci Catheter-Related Bacteremia Without Complication

In patients with methicillin-resistant coagulase-negative staphylococci catheter-related bacteremia without complication, the physician may retain the catheter and use: (i) vancomycin therapy administered through a peripheral catheter for 10-14 days; and (ii) antibiotic lock therapy for 10-14 days. Antibiotic lock therapy involves instillation of a highly concentrated antibiotic solution into an intravascular catheter lumen for the purpose of bacterial eradication, in patients for whom catheter salvage is the goal [36, 37, 38, 39]. In methicillin-resistant coagulase-negative staphylococci, gentamicin or vancomycin could be used as lock therapy. It has to be always used in combination with systemic vancomycin. For vancomycin lock therapy, vancomycin is combined with heparin and instilled with high concentration (2.5 to 5 mg/mL i.e > 1000 times the MIC of the microorganism) and in sufficient volume to fill each catheter lumen (usually 2-5 mL), each day during 10 to 14 days [36, 40]. If blood cultures remain positive 72 h after the initiation of appropriate therapy, the catheter should be removed. For some authors, the duration of the therapy should be prolonged 4 to 6 weeks in uncomplicated *S. aureus* bacteremia, especially if patients have diabetes, if they are immunosuppressed (i.e, if they received immunosuppressive drugs including corticosteroids or if they are neutropenic) [36].

Complicated Catheter-Related Bacteremia

In patients with complicated catheter-related bacteremia, the catheter has to be removed, and the duration of the vancomycin therapy has to be prolonged to 4 to 6 weeks, with the optional addition of gentamicin (3 mg/kg/day) for the first 3-5 days of therapy, as it has been described for patients with native valve endocarditis [21, 26, 27, 41].

Methicillin-Resistant Staphylococci Endocarditis

Methicillin-resistant staphylococci could be responsible for endocarditis. The standard dose of 30 mg/kg/day is usually recommended in endocarditis, but some authors advise high trough serum vancomycin concentrations (25-30 mg/L), even if patients with endocarditis are at high risk of kidney injury [27]. In all cases of staphylococcal endocarditis, early evaluation for valve replacement surgery is recommended [43, 44].

Native Valve Endocarditis

Native valve endocarditis (i.e in a patient without prosthetic valve) is mainly due to streptococci or *S. aureus*. In patients with MRSA native valve endocarditis, vancomycin remains the drug of choice, at a daily dose of 30 mg/kg in 2 to 4 injections, for 4 to 6 weeks. Vancomycin should be used in combination with gentamicin (3 mg/kg/day) for the first 3-5 days of therapy, although the clinical benefit of the addition of gentamicin has not been clearly demonstrated (but drug combination, by its synergic effect, enhances bactericidal activity) [6, 21, 26, 27, 41].

Prosthetic Valve Endocarditis

Both MRSA and methicillin-resistant coagulase-negative staphylococci could be involved in prosthetic valve endocarditis.

As these pathogens are difficult to eradicate, vancomycin has to be combined with gentamicin during the first 14 days, and with rifampin during 6 weeks [21, 27, 41, 45].

Conclusion

Vancomycin remains the drug of choice in patients with methicillin-resistant *S. aureus* or coagulase-negative staphylococci bacteremia, catheter-related bacteremia or endocarditis. The management of such infections, the duration of vancomycin therapy and the duration of the companion drug, depend mainly on patient's clinical evaluation at baseline and during vancomycin therapy.

References

[1]   Ferry, T.; Perpoint, T.; Vandenesch, F. Etienne J. Virulence determinants in Staphylococcus aureus and their involvement in clinical syndromes. *Curr. Infect. Dis. Rep.* 2005 Nov; 7(6): 420-8.

[2]   Miragaia, M.; Couto, I.; Pereira, S. F. F.; Kristinsson, K. G.; Westh, H.; Jarlov, J.O. et al. Molecular Characterization of Methicillin-Resistant Staphylococcus epidermidis Clones: Evidence of Geographic Dissemination. *J. Clin. Microbiol.* févr 2002; 40(2): 430-438.

[3]   Cosgrove, S. E.; Sakoulas, G.; Perencevich, E. N.; Schwaber, M. J.; Karchmer, A. W.; Carmeli, Y. Comparison of mortality associated with methicillin-resistant and methicillin-susceptible Staphylococcus aureus bacteremia: a meta-analysis. *Clin. Infect. Dis. Off. Publ. Infect. Dis. Soc. Am.* 1 janv 2003; 36(1): 53-59.

[4]   Whitby, M.; McLaws, M. L.; Berry, G. Risk of death from methicillin-resistant Staphylococcus aureus bacteraemia: a meta-analysis. *Med. J. Aust.* 3 sept 2001; 175(5): 264-267.

[5]   Tristan, A.; Ferry, T.; Durand, G.; Dauwalder, O.; Bes, M.; Lina, G.; Vandenesch, F.; Etienne, J. Virulence determinants in community and hospital meticillin-resistant Staphylococcus aureus. *J. Hosp. Infect.* 2007 Jun; 65 Suppl 2:105-9.

[6]   Garau, J.; Bouza, E.; Chastre, J.; Gudiol, F.; Harbarth, S. Management of methicillin-resistant Staphylococcus aureus infections. *Clin. Microbiol. Infect.* 2009; 15(2): 125-36.

[7]   Mohr, J. F.; Murray, B. E.; Point: Vancomycin Is Not Obsolete for the Treatment of Infection Caused by Methicillin-Resistant Staphylococcus aureus. *Clin. Infect. Dis.* 15 juin 2007; 44(12): 1536-1542.

[8]   Kropec, A.; Daschner, F. D. Penetration into tissues of various drugs active against Gram-positive bacteria. *J. Antimicrob. Chemother.* 1 janv 1991; 27(suppl B): 9-15.

[9]   Cruciani, M.; Gatti, G.; Lazzarini, L.; Furlan, G.; Broccali, G.; Malena, M. et al. Penetration of vancomycin into human lung tissue. *J. Antimicrob. Chemother.* 11 janv 1996; 38(5): 865-869.

[10] Clinical and Laboratory Standards Institute, Wayne P. Clinical and Laboratory Standards Institute; 2007. *Performance standars for antimicrobial susceptibility testing; seventeenth informational supplement.* 2007; Standard M100-S17.

[11] Lodise, T. P.; Graves, J.; Evans, A.; Graffunder, E.; Helmecke, M.; Lomaestro, B. M. et al. Relationship between Vancomycin MIC and Failure among Patients with Methicillin-Resistant Staphylococcus aureus Bacteremia Treated with Vancomycin. *Antimicrob. Agents Chemother.* 9 janv 2008; 52(9): 3315-3320.

[12] Sakoulas, G.; Moise-Broder, P. A.; Schentag, J.; Forrest, A.; Moellering, R. C.; Eliopoulos, G. M. Relationship of MIC and Bactericidal Activity to Efficacy of Vancomycin for Treatment of Methicillin-Resistant Staphylococcus aureus Bacteremia. *J. Clin. Microbiol.* 6 janv 2004; 42(6): 2398-2402.

[13] Soriano, A.; Marco, F.; Martínez, J. A.; Pisos, E.; Almela, M.; Dimova, V. P. et al. Influence of Vancomycin Minimum Inhibitory Concentration on the Treatment of Methicillin-Resistant Staphylococcus aureus Bacteremia. *Clin. Infect. Dis.* 15 janv 2008; 46(2): 193-200.

[14] Hiramatsu, K. Vancomycin-resistant Staphylococcus aureus: a new model of antibiotic resistance. *Lancet Infect. Dis.* oct 2001; 1(3): 147-155.

[15] Reduced susceptibility of Staphylococcus aureus to vancomycin--Japan, 1996. *Mmwr Morb. Mortal. Wkly. Rep.* 11 juill 1997; 46(27): 624-626.

[16] Kollef, M. H. Limitations of Vancomycin in the Management of Resistant Staphylococcal Infections. *Clin. Infect. Dis.* 15 sept 2007; 45(Supplement 3): S191-S195.

[17] Charles, P. G. P.; Ward, P. B.; Johnson, P. D. R.; Howden, B. P.; Grayson, M. L. Clinical Features Associated with Bacteremia Due to Heterogeneous Vancomycin-Intermediate Staphylococcus aureus. *Clin. Infect. Dis.* 2 janv 2004; 38(3): 448-451.

[18] Dudley, M.; Griffith, E.; Corcoran, C. et al. Program and Abstracts of the 39th Interscience Conference of Antimicrobial Agents and Chemotherapy□ : *Pharmacokinetic-pharmacodynamic indices for vancomycin treatment of susceptible intermediate S. aureus in the neutropenic murine thigh model* [abstract 2031]. San Francisco, CA; 1999.

[19] Moise-Broder, P. A.; Forrest, A.; Birmingham, M. C.; Schentag, D. J. J. Pharmacodynamics of Vancomycin and Other Antimicrobials in Patients with Staphylococcus aureus Lower Respiratory Tract Infections. *Clin. Pharmacokinet.* 1 nov 2004; 43(13): 925-942.

[20] Jeffres, M. N.; Isakow, W.; Doherty, J. A. et al. Predictors of mortality for methicillin-resistant Staphylococcus aureus health-care-associated pneumonia: specific evaluation of vancomycin pharmacokinetic indices. *Chest*. 2006 Oct; 130(4): 947-55.

[21] Liu, C.; Bayer, A.; Cosgrove, S. E.; Daum, R. S.; Fridkin, S. K.; Gorwitz, R. J. et al. Clinical Practice Guidelines by the Infectious Diseases Society of America for the Treatment of Methicillin-Resistant Staphylococcus aureus Infections in Adults and Children: Executive Summary. *Clin. Infect. Dis.* 2 janv 2011; 52(3): 285-292.

[22] Cosgrove, S.; Fowler, V. Optimizing Therapy for Methicillin-resistant Staphylococcus aureus Bacteremia. *Semin. Respir. Crit. Care Med.* déc 2007; 28(6): 624-631.

[23] James, J. K.; Palmer, S. M.; Levine, D. P.; Rybak, M. J. Comparison of conventional dosing versus continuous-infusion vancomycin therapy for patients with suspected or documented gram-positive infections. Antimicrob. *Agents Chemother.* 3 janv 1996; 40(3): 696-700.

[24] Lacy, M. K.; Tessier, P. Nicolau, D. P.; Nightingale, C. H.; Quintiliani, R. Comparison of vancomycin pharmacodynamics (1 g every 12 or 24 h) against methicillin-resistant staphylococci. *Int. J. Antimicrob. Agents.* juin 2000; 15(1): 25-30.

[25] Boucher, H.; Miller, L. G. ; Razonable, R. R. Serious Infections Caused by Methicillin-Resistant Staphylococcus aureus. *Clin. Infect. Dis.* 15 sept 2010; 51(S2): S183-S197.

[26] Gould, F. K.; Denning, D. W.; Elliott, T. S. J.; Foweraker, J.; Perry, J. D.; Prendergast, B. D. et al. Guidelines for the diagnosis and antibiotic

treatment of endocarditis in adults: a report of the Working Party of the British Society for Antimicrobial Chemotherapy. *J. Antimicrob. Chemother.* 14 nov 2011; 67(2): 269-289.

[27] Endorsed by the European Society of Clinical Microbiology and Infectious Diseases (ESCMID) and by the International Society of Chemotherapy (ISC) for Infection and Cancer, Authors/Task Force Members, Habib, G.; Hoen, B.; Tornos, P.; Thuny, F. et al. Guidelines on the prevention, diagnosis, and treatment of infective endocarditis (new version 2009): The Task Force on the Prevention, Diagnosis, and Treatment of Infective Endocarditis of the European Society of Cardiology (ESC). *Eur. Heart J.* 27 août 2009; 30(19): 2369-2413.

[28] Raad, II.; Sabbagh, M. F. Optimal duration of therapy for catheter-related Staphylococcus aureus bacteremia: a study of 55 cases and review. *Clin. Infect. Dis. Off. Publ. Infect. Dis. Soc. Am.* janv 1992; 14(1): 75-82.

[29] Malanoski, G. J.; Samore, M. H.; Pefanis, A.; Karchmer, A. W. Staphylococcus aureus catheter-associated bacteremia. Minimal effective therapy and unusual infectious complications associated with arterial sheath catheters. *Arch. Intern. Med.* 12 juin 1995; 155(11): 1161-1166.

[30] Ehni, W. F.; Reller, L. B. Short-course therapy for catheter-associated Staphylococcus aureus bacteremia. *Arch. Intern. Med.* mars 1989; 149(3): 533-536.

[31] Jernigan, J. A.; Farr, B. M. Short-course therapy of catheter-related Staphylococcus aureus bacteremia: a meta-analysis. *Ann. Intern. Med.* 15 août 1993; 119(4): 304-311.

[32] Cosgrove, S. E.; Fowler, Jr. V. G. Management of Methicillin-Resistant Staphylococcus aureus Bacteremia. *Clin. Infect. Dis.* juin 2008; 46(S5): S386-S393.

[33] Fowler, V. G. Jr.; Li, J.; Corey, G. R.; Boley, J.; Marr, K. A.; Gopal, A. K. et al. Role of echocardiography in evaluation of patients with Staphylococcus aureus bacteremia: experience in 103 patients. *J. Am. Coll. Cardiol.* oct 1997; 30(4): 1072-1078.

[34] Sullenberger, A. L.; Avedissian, L. S.; Kent, S. M. Importance of transesophageal echocardiography in the evaluation of Staphylococcus aureus bacteremia. *J. Heart Valve Dis.* janv 2005; 14(1): 23-28.

[35] Rosen, A. B.; Fowler, V. G. Jr.; Corey, G. R.; Downs, S. M.; Biddle, A. K.; Li, J. et al. Cost-effectiveness of transesophageal echocardiography to determine the duration of therapy for intravascular catheter-associated

Staphylococcus aureus bacteremia. *Ann. Intern. Med.* 18 mai 1999; 130(10): 810-820.

[36] Mermel, L. A.; Allon, M.; Bouza, E.; Craven, D. E.; Flynn P, O'Grady NP, et al. Clinical Practice Guidelines for the Diagnosis and Management of Intravascular Catheter-Related Infection: 2009 Update by the Infectious Diseases Society of America. *Clin. Infect. Dis.* 7 janv 2009; 49(1): 1-45.

[37] Fernandez-Hidalgo, N.; Almirante, B.; Calleja, R.; Ruiz, I.; Planes, A. M.; Rodriguez, D. et al. Antibiotic-lock therapy for long-term intravascular catheter-related bacteraemia: results of an open, non-comparative study. *J. Antimicrob. Chemother.* 6 janv 2006; 57(6): 1172-1180.

[38] Fortún, J.; Grill, F.; Martín-Dávila, P.; Blázquez, J.; Tato, M.; Sánchez-Corral, J. et al. Treatment of long-term intravascular catheter-related bacteraemia with antibiotic-lock therapy. *J. Antimicrob. Chemother.* 10 janv 2006; 58(4): 816-821.

[39] Fowler, V. G.; Justice, A.; Moore, C.; Benjamin, D. K.; Woods, C. W.; Campbell, S. et al. Risk Factors For Hematogenous Complications of Intravascular Catheter—Associated Staphylococcus aureus Bacteremia. *Clin. Infect. Dis.* 3 janv 2005; 40(5): 695-703.

[40] Soriano, A.; Bregada, E.; Marqués, J. M.; Ortega, M.; Bové, A.; Martínez, J. A et al. Decreasing gradient of antibiotic concentration in the lumen of catheters locked with vancomycin. *Eur. J. Clin. Microbiol. Infect. Dis. Off. Publ. Eur. Soc. Clin. Microbiol.* sept 2007; 26(9): 659-661.

[41] Baddour, L. M.; Wilson, W. R.; Bayer, A. S.; Fowler, V. G.; Bolger, A. F.; Levison, M. E. et al. Infective Endocarditis Diagnosis, Antimicrobial Therapy, and Management of Complications: A Statement for Healthcare Professionals From the Committee on Rheumatic Fever, Endocarditis, and Kawasaki Disease, Council on Cardiovascular Disease in the Young, and the Councils on Clinical Cardiology, Stroke, and Cardiovascular Surgery and Anesthesia, American Heart Association: Endorsed by the Infectious Diseases Society of America. *Circulation.* 14 juin 2005; 111(23): e394-e434.

[42] Kang, D-H.; Kim, Y-J.; Kim, S-H.; Sun, B. J.; Kim, D-H.; Yun, S-C. et al. Early surgery versus conventional treatment for infective endocarditis. *N. Engl. J. Med.* 28 juin 2012; 366(26): 2466-2473.

[43] Barsic, B.; Dickerman, S.; Krajinovic, V.; Pappas, P.; Altclas, J.; Carosi, G. et al. Influence of the timing of cardiac surgery on the outcome of

patients with infective endocarditis and stroke. *Clin. Infect. Dis. Off. Publ. Infect. Dis. Soc. Am.* janv 2013; 56(2): 209-217.

[44] Cabell, C. H.; Abrutyn, E.; Fowler, V. G. Jr.; Hoen, B.; Miro, J. M.; Corey, G. R. et al. Use of surgery in patients with native valve infective endocarditis: results from the International Collaboration on Endocarditis Merged Database. *Am. Heart J.* nov 2005; 150(5): 1092-1098.

[45] Perlroth, J.; Kuo, M.; Tan, J.; Bayer, A. S.; Miller, L. G. Adjunctive use of rifampin for the treatment of Staphylococcus aureus infections: a systematic review of the literature. *Arch. Intern. Med.* 28 avr 2008; 168(8): 805-819.

In: Vancomycin
Editor: Abu Gafar Hossion

ISBN: 978-1-62948-559-1
© 2013 Nova Science Publishers, Inc.

Chapter 7

Clinical Use of Vancomycin in MRSA Ventilator-Associated Pneumonia

Nader Chebib[1], Agathe Sénéchal[1,2],
Jean-Christophe Richard[2,3], Claire Tissot[1],
Alicia Marquet[1], Judith Karsenty[1,2],
Florence Ader[1,2,3], Christian Chidiac[1,2,3]
and Tristan Ferry[1,2,3,*

[1]Infectious diseases department, Croix-Rousse Hospital,
Hospices Civils de Lyon, France
[2]Claude Bernard University, Lyon, France
[3]Intensive Care Unit, Croix-Rousse Hospital,
Hospices Civils de Lyon, France
[4]Centre International de Recherche en Infectiologie, CIRI, Inserm U1111,
CNRS UMR5308, ENS de Lyon, UCBL1, Lyon, France

* Corresponding author: Tristan Ferry – Infectious Diseases department, Croix-rousse Hospital, 103 Grande-Rue de la Croix-Rousse, 69004 Lyon, France. Email: tristan.ferry@univ-lyon1.fr.

Abstract

We have developed here the clinical use of vancomycin in MRSA hospital-acquired pneumonia. MRSA hospital-acquired pneumonia is associated with a significant morbidity and long hospital stays, particularly in intensive care units for patients with ventilator-associated pneumonia (VAP). Patients with VAP should have vancomycin as empirical therapy, immediately after the bronchoalveolar lavage, if MRSA is suspected (patient known to be MRSA carrier, late VAP). Vancomycin has to be administered intravenously through a central venous catheter with a dosage of 15 mg/kg/d twice a day. The dose has to be reduced for patients with renal failure. Monitoring serum concentration is required to optimize vancomycin therapy. Linezolid may be more effective than vancomycin, as suggested by two randomized controlled double-blind trials, as a possible consequence of vancomycin poor penetration into the lung. Linezolid could also be used to terminate the therapy in patients treated with vancomycin for MRSA VAP, if the central venous catheter is lost. Two weeks of therapy are usually sufficient to treat MRSA VAP.

Keywords: Vancomycin, MRSA, ventilator-associated pneumonia, linezolid

Introduction

Ventilator associated pneumonia (VAP) is a subtype of hospital-acquired pneumonia which also includes healthcare-associated pneumonia (occurs in patients with recent close contact with the health care system) and nosocomial pneumonia (occurs in hospitalized patients, at least 48-72 hours after admission).

VAP occurs in patients who are receiving mechanical ventilation in intensive care units. The diagnosis and treatment of VAP is of crucial importance, as VAP is associated with a significant morbidity, in-hospital mortality, and long hospital stay, especially if methicillin-resistant *S. aureus* (MRSA) is involved. VAP diagnosis requires an association of clinical, biological, radiological, and microbiological signs occurring in a patient after at least 48 hours of mechanical ventilation, among the followings: new or progressive radiologic opacities; fever > 38°C; leukopenia < 4000/mm^3 or leukocytosis > 12000/mm^3; purulent or increased sputum and respiratory secretions; dyspnea or cough; worsening gas exchange and increased oxygen requirements; direct identification of a microbiological agent in the respiratory tract, with different thresholds according to the diagnostic technique used (e.g 10^4 UFC/mL for broncho-alveolar lavage, 10^6 UFC/mL for unprotected bronchial aspirates); or alternative methods such as positive blood cultures, positive pleural fluid, or lung biopsy [1, 2].

The aim of this chapter was to review the clinical use of vancomycin in patients with VAP due to MRSA.

Epidemiology

VAP ranks among the most frequent healthcare associated infections, and even comes first in the intensive care units (ICU) [1, 3]. Its incidence ranges from 6% to 68% depending on the time and geographic setting of epidemiologic studies, as well as the nature of the ICU [4, 5, 67]. VAP may be caused by a wide spectrum of bacterial pathogens, but *Staphyloccus aureus* (SA) is one of the most commonly found agents, with an incidence ranging from 16% to 33%. Meticillin resistant *Staphyloccus aureus* (MRSA) represents 33% to 77,5% of SA isolated cultures [7, 8, 9, 10, 11, 12], and is more frequent in late-onset VAP (occurring more than 4 days after the start of mechanical ventilation) [13], as well as in neurological and surgical ICUs [9, 14].

Risk Factors

The main route for SA VAP is repetitive micro-aspiration of bacteria colonizing the oropharynx and the gastric mucosa. Other routes of infection include direct aerial inhalation, hematological diffusion, and infection by contiguity.

Several risk factors for SA VAP have been identified and include: advanced age [1, 9, 15, 16], male sex (16, 17), comorbidities (especially diabetes mellitus) [1, 15, 16], nasal and tracheal colonization by SA [1, 18, 19)], prolonged mechanical ventilation and ICU stay (1, 4, 20-25), coma and cerebral trauma [17, 18, 19], as well as prior use of antibiotics, notably the fluoroquinolones [1, 5, 26, 27].

Morbidity/Mortality/Cost

MRSA VAPs are responsible for an increased morbidity and mortality, as well as economic costs. They have been shown to expand mechanical ventilation duration, hospital and ICU length of stay [1, 17, 28]. Mortality remains high despite antibiotic use, varying from 30% to 70% and it is even more important in patients with SA bacteremia [9, 29, 30, 31, 32].

Treatment

Glycopeptides and more precisely vancomycin, have long been the gold-standard treatment of MRSA VAP, even though its pharmacokinetic profile may be suboptimal in pulmonary infections. Penetration of vancomycin into lung compartments is relatively poor. Its concentration in epithelial lining fluid does not exceed 20% of the plasma levels, with high interindividual and intraindividual variations resulting in inadequate concentrations [33]. This could partially explain the high rate of clinical failure reported, mounting up to 40% in certain studies [1, 34, 35].

In 2003, a post-hoc analysis of 2 prospective double blind trials, conducted in 160 patients comparing linezolid to vancomycin, each associated to aztreonam, found significantly better survival (80% vs. 64%) and cure rates (59% vs. 36%) with linezolid [36, 37, 38]. However, this study was subject to several methodological critics (retrospective analysis and insufficient vancomycin dosage), and other trials were subsequently made. A meta-analysis published in 2011, included 8 randomized controlled trials (RCT) from 2001 to 2008, comparing glycopeptides to linezolid, in 1641 patients [39]. Six RCT tested vancomycin and the remaining 2 tested teicoplanin. There was no significant difference in the primary end point which was the rate of clinical success (RR 1.04 CI 95%, 0.97-1.11; $p = 0.28$), regardless of the type of glycopeptides. There was no difference as well in mortality rates and microbiologic success. In 2012, a multicentric RCT named Zephyr compared vancomycin (15 mg/Kg/12hours) to linezolid (600 mg/12hours) in patients with MRSA pneumonia. Clinical outcome was evaluated in 2 cohorts: the modified intention to treat group (mITT) with 448 patients, and the per-protocol group (PP) with 348 patients [40]. In the PP population, 57.6% of patients treated with linezolid attained clinical success, compared to 46.6% of patients treated with vancomycin ($p = 0.042$, CI 95% 0.5-21.6). All-cause 60-

day mortality did not differ in the ITT and mITT populations. This study has several limitations, including the imperfect initial comparability of the 2 groups (more mechanically ventilated patients, more patients with personal history of kidney failure, and more SARM bacteremia in the vancomycin group), the large confidence interval shown in the clinical response, the number of patients with infratherapeutic blood level of vancomycin, the lack of vancomycin loading dose and the number of patients excluded from the analysis [41].

American and European guidelines concerning the treatment of MRSA VAP, do not privilege the use of one antibiotic over the other, and recommend the use of either intravenous vancomycin 15-20 mg/Kg/12 hours or 1 g/12 hours, or linezolid 600 mg/12 hours. The trough level recommended for vancomycin is 15-20 mg/L [1, 13, 42]. Once the causal agent identified, combination therapy directed at MRSA is not recommended [1].

The use of continuous vancomycin infusion has not shown higher efficiency compared to discontinuous infusion [1]. A meta-analysis of 1 RCT and 5 observational studies, not limited to pulmonary infections, did not find a difference in overall mortality, but a significant lower risk of nephrotoxicity with continuous infusion of vancomycin [43, 44].

Several studies have found that vancomycin serum concentrations are often too low, mainly because vancomycin distribution volume is increased in critically ill patients. Hence, when using continuous infusion, a loading dose of vancomycin 25-30mg/Kg [45], up to 35 mg/kg [46] delivered over 1 hour, is essential to achieve adequate therapeutic concentrations rapidly. The impact of this strategy on clinical outcome is still unknown, and it figures in the American guidelines with a grade B and a level of proof amounting to 3.

The recommended traditional duration of antibiotic therapy is 7 to 21 days, with an emphasis on reducing this duration to as short as 7 days when the initial empiric antibiotherapy is appropriate, with several studies not showing any worse outcome when shorter courses are used [1, 47]. A multicenter, prospective, parallel-group, open-label RCT named Prorata, compared a procalcitonin-guided strategy to start and stop antibiotics in non-surgical intensive care patients with suspected bacterial infections [48], with a control group in which antibiotics were administered according to international guidelines.

When procalcitonin concentration was less than 80% of the peak concentration, or had reached an absolute concentration of less than 0,5 µg/L, investigators were encouraged to discontinue antibiotics. In the procalcitonin group, 183 out of 307 patients (79%) had a pulmonary infection, out of which

66 (22%) had VAP. No significant difference in 28-day and 60-day mortality was shown, as well as in relapse or superinfection percentage, but patients in the procalcitonin group had significantly more days without antibiotics than did those in the control group (absolute difference of 2.7 days). Whether those results apply to MRSA VAP remains however unknown, since this specific subgroup was not reported.

Conclusion

Vancomycin holds a central place in the treatment of MRSA VAP despite the arrival of other agents such as linezolid. The physician's choice should be based on individual patient data, with a special consideration to the risk of nephrotoxicity with vancomycin (especially when combined with aminoglycosides), and to the resistance profile of MRSA as shown by its CMI to vancomycin. Blood levels of vancomycin should be monitored daily, and doses should be adapted if necessary, in order to maximize chances of clinical success and diminish the risk of renal failure.

References

[1]   "Guidelines for the management of adults with hospital-acquired, ventilator-associated, and healthcare-associated pneumonia," *Am. J. Respir. Crit. Care Med.*, vol. 171, no. 4, pp. 388–416, Feb. 2005.

[2]   Garner, J. S.; Jarvis, W. R.; Emori, T. G.; Horan, T. C. and Hughes, J. M. "CDC definitions for nosocomial infections, 1988," *Am. J. Infect. Control*, vol. 16, no. 3, pp. 128–140, Jun. 1988.

[3]   Safdar, N.; Dezfulian, C.; Collard, H. R. and Saint, S. "Clinical and economic consequences of ventilator-associated pneumonia: a systematic review," *Crit. Care Med.*, vol. 33, no. 10, pp. 2184–2193, Oct. 2005.

[4]   Chastre, J. and Fagon, J.-Y. "Ventilator-associated pneumonia," *Am. J. Respir. Crit. Care Med.*, vol. 165, no. 7, pp. 867–903, Apr. 2002.

[5]   Rello, J. and Diaz, E. "Pneumonia in the intensive care unit," *Crit. Care Med.*, vol. 31, no. 10, pp. 2544–2551, Oct. 2003.

[6]   Vincent, J. L.; Bihari, D. J.; Suter, P. M.; Bruining, H. A.; White, J.; Nicolas-Chanoin, M. H.; Wolff, M.; Spencer, R. C. and Hemmer, M.

"The prevalence of nosocomial infection in intensive care units in Europe. Results of the European Prevalence of Infection in Intensive Care (EPIC) Study. EPIC International Advisory Committee," *Jama J. Am. Med. Assoc.*, vol. 274, no. 8, pp. 639–644, Aug. 1995.

[7]   Vincent, J.-L.; Rello, J.; Marshall, J.; Silva, E.; Anzueto, A.; Martin, C. D.; Moreno, R.; Lipman, J.; Gomersall, C.; Sakr, Y.; and Reinhart, K. "International study of the prevalence and outcomes of infection in intensive care units," *Jama J. Am. Med. Assoc.*, vol. 302, no. 21, pp. 2323–2329, Dec. 2009.

[8]   Koulenti, D.; Lisboa, T.; Brun-Buisson, C. ; Krueger, W.; Macor, A.; Sole-Violan, J.; Diaz, E.; Topeli, A.; DeWaele, J.; Carneiro, A.; Martin-Loeches, I.; Armaganidis, A. and Rello, J. "Spectrum of practice in the diagnosis of nosocomial pneumonia in patients requiring mechanical ventilation in European intensive care units," *Crit. Care Med.*, vol. 37, no. 8, pp. 2360–2368, Aug. 2009.

[9]   Meyer, E.; Schwab, F. and Gastmeier, P. "Nosocomial methicillin resistant Staphylococcus aureus pneumonia - epidemiology and trends based on data of a network of 586 German ICUs (2005-2009)," *Eur. J. Med. Res.*, vol. 15, no. 12, pp. 514–524, Nov. 2010.

[10] Hidron, A. I.; Edwards, J. R.; Patel, J.; Horan, T. C.; Sievert, D. M.; Pollock, D. A. and Fridkin, S. K. "NHSN annual update: antimicrobial-resistant pathogens associated with healthcare-associated infections: annual summary of data reported to the National Healthcare Safety Network at the Centers for Disease Control and Prevention, 2006-2007," *Infect. Control Hosp. Epidemiol. Off. J. Soc. Hosp. Epidemiol. Am.*, vol. 29, no. 11, pp. 996–1011, Nov. 2008.

[11] Rosenthal, V. D.; Maki, D. G.; Jamulitrat, S.; Medeiros, E. A.; Todi, S. K.; Gomez, D. Y. Leblebicioglu, H.; Abu Khader, I.; Miranda Novales, M. G.; Berba, R.; Ramírez Wong, F. M.; Barkat, A.; Pino, O. R.; Dueñas, L.; Mitrev, Z.; Bijie, H.; Gurskis, V.; Kanj, S. S.; Mapp, T.; Hidalgo, R. F.; Ben Jaballah, N.; Raka, L.; Gikas, A.; Ahmed, A.; Thu, L. T. A. and Guzmán Siritt, M. E. "International Nosocomial Infection Control Consortium (INICC) report, data summary for 2003-2008, issued June 2009," *Am. J. Infect. Control*, vol. 38, no. 2, pp. 95–104.e2, Mar. 2010.

[12] Rello, J.; Molano, D.; Villabon, M.; Reina, R.; Rita-Quispe, R.; Previgliano, I.; Afonso, E.; and Restrepo, M. I. "Differences in hospital- and ventilator-associated pneumonia due to Staphylococcus aureus (methicillin-susceptible and methicillin-resistant) between Europe and

Latin America: A comparison of the EUVAP and LATINVAP study cohorts," *Med. Intensiva Soc. Espanola Med. Intensiva Unidades Coronarias*, Jun. 2012.

[13] Torres, A.; Ewig, S.; Lode, H.; Carlet, J. For The European HAP working group, "Defining, treating and preventing hospital acquired pneumonia: European perspective," *Intensive Care Med.*, vol. 35, no. 1, pp. 9–29, Nov. 2008.

[14] Campbell, W.; Hendrix, E.; Schwalbe, R.; Fattom, A. and Edelman, R. "Head-injured patients who are nasal carriers of Staphylococcus aureus are at high risk for Staphylococcus aureus pneumonia," *Crit. Care Med.*, vol. 27, no. 4, pp. 798–801, Apr. 1999.

[15] Haque, N. Z.; Arshad, S.; Peyrani, P.; Ford, K. D.; Perri, M. B.; Jacobsen, G.; Reyes, K.; Scerpella, E. G.; Ramirez, J. A. and Zervos, M. J. "Analysis of pathogen and host factors related to clinical outcomes in patients with hospital-acquired pneumonia due to methicillin-resistant Staphylococcus aureus," *J. Clin. Microbiol.*, vol. 50, no. 5, pp. 1640–1644, May 2012.

[16] Kofteridis, D. P.; Papadakis, J. A.; Bouros, D.; Nikolaides, P.; Kioumis, G.; Levidiotou, S.; Maltezos, E.; Kastanakis, S.; Kartali, S. and Gikas, A. "Nosocomial lower respiratory tract infections: prevalence and risk factors in 14 Greek hospitals," *Eur. J. Clin. Microbiol. Infect. Dis.*, Nov. 2004.

[17] Rello, J.; Ollendorf, D. A.; Oster, G.; Vera-Llonch, M.; Bellm, L.; Redman, R.; and Kollef, M. H. "Epidemiology and outcomes of ventilator-associated pneumonia in a large US database," *Chest*, vol. 122, no. 6, pp. 2115–2121, Dec. 2002.

[18] Pujol, M.; Corbella, X.; Peña, C.; Pallares, R.; Dorca, J.; Verdaguer, R.; Diaz-Prieto, A.; Ariza, J.; and Gudiol, F. "Clinical and epidemiological findings in mechanically-ventilated patients with methicillin-resistant Staphylococcus aureus pneumonia," *Eur. J. Clin. Microbiol. Infect. Dis. Off. Publ. Eur. Soc. Clin. Microbiol.*, vol. 17, no. 9, pp. 622–628, Sep. 1998.

[19] George, D. L.; Falk, P. S.; Wunderink, R. G.; Leeper Jr, K. V.; Meduri, G. U.; Steere, E. L.; Corbett, C. E. and Mayhall, C. G. "Epidemiology of ventilator-acquired pneumonia based on protected bronchoscopic sampling," *Am. J. Respir. Crit. Care Med.*, vol. 158, no. 6, pp. 1839–1847, Dec. 1998.

[20] Asensio, A.; Guerrero, A.; Quereda, C.; Lizán, M. and Martinez-Ferrer, M. "Colonization and infection with methicillin-resistant

Staphylococcus aureus: associated factors and eradication," *Infect. Control Hosp. Epidemiol. Off. J. Soc. Hosp. Epidemiol. Am.*, vol. 17, no. 1, pp. 20–28, Jan. 1996.

[21] Graffunder, E. M. and Venezia, R. A. "Risk factors associated with nosocomial methicillin-resistant Staphylococcus aureus (MRSA) infection including previous use of antimicrobials," *J. Antimicrob. Chemother.*, vol. 49, no. 6, pp. 999–1005, Jun. 2002.

[22] Celis, R.; Torres, A.; Gatell, J. M.; Almela, M.; Rodríguez-Roisin, R. and Agustí-Vidal, A. "Nosocomial pneumonia. A multivariate analysis of risk and prognosis," *Chest*, vol. 93, no. 2, pp. 318–324, Feb. 1988.

[23] Torres, A.; Aznar, R.; Gatell, J. M.; Jiménez, P.; González, J.; Ferrer, A.; Celis, R. and Rodriguez-Roisin, R. "Incidence, risk, and prognosis factors of nosocomial pneumonia in mechanically ventilated patients," *Am. Rev. Respir. Dis.*, vol. 142, no. 3, pp. 523–528, Sep. 1990.

[24] Craven, D. E. and Steger, K. A. "Nosocomial pneumonia in mechanically ventilated adult patients: epidemiology and prevention in 1996," *Semin. Respir. Infect.*, vol. 11, no. 1, pp. 32–53, Mar. 1996.

[25] Horan, T. C.; Culver, D. H.; Gaynes, R. P.; Jarvis, W. R.; Edwards, J. R. and Reid, C. R. "Nosocomial infections in surgical patients in the United States, January 1986-June 1992. National Nosocomial Infections Surveillance (NNIS) System," *Infect. Control Hosp. Epidemiol. Off. J. Soc. Hosp. Epidemiol. Am.*, vol. 14, no. 2, pp. 73–80, Feb. 1993.

[26] Monnet, D. L. and Frimodt-Møller, N. "Antimicrobial-drug use and methicillin-resistant Staphylococcus aureus," *Emerg. Infect. Dis.*, vol. 7, no. 1, pp. 161–163, Feb. 2001.

[27] Manhold, C.; von Rolbicki, U.; Brase, R.; Timm, J.; von Pritzbuer, E.; Heimesaat, M. and Kljucar, S. "Outbreaks of Staphylococcus aureus infections during treatment of late onset pneumonia with ciprofloxacin in a prospective, randomized study," *Intensive Care Med.*, vol. 24, no. 12, pp. 1327–1330, Dec. 1998.

[28] Hugonnet, S.; Eggimann, P.; Borst, F.; Maricot, P.; Chevrolet, J.-C. and Pittet, D. "Impact of ventilator-associated pneumonia on resource utilization and patient outcome," *Infect. Control Hosp. Epidemiol. Off. J. Soc. Hosp. Epidemiol. Am.*, vol. 25, no. 12, pp. 1090–1096, Dec. 2004.

[29] Cosgrove, S. E.; Sakoulas, G.; Perencevich, E. N.; Schwaber, M. J.; Karchmer, A. W. and Carmeli, Y. "Comparison of mortality associated with methicillin-resistant and methicillin-susceptible Staphylococcus aureus bacteremia: a meta-analysis," *Clin. Infect. Dis. Off. Publ. Infect. Dis. Soc. Am.*, vol. 36, no. 1, pp. 53–59, Jan. 2003.

[30] Whitby, M.; McLaws, M. L. and Berry, G. "Risk of death from methicillin-resistant Staphylococcus aureus bacteraemia: a meta-analysis," *Med. J. Aust.*, vol. 175, no. 5, pp. 264–267, Sep. 2001.

[31] Shorr, A. F.; Tabak, Y. P.; Gupta, V.; Johannes, R. S.; Liu, L. Z. and Kollef, M. H. "Morbidity and cost burden of methicillin-resistant Staphylococcus aureus in early onset ventilator-associated pneumonia," *Crit. Care Lond. Engl.*, vol. 10, no. 3, p. R97, 2006.

[32] González, C.; Rubio, M.; Romero-Vivas, J.; González, M. and Picazo, J. J. "Staphylococcus aureus bacteremic pneumonia: differences between community and nosocomial acquisition," *Int. J. Infect. Dis. Ijid Off. Publ. Int. Soc. Infect. Dis.*, vol. 7, no. 2, pp. 102–108, Jun. 2003.

[33] Lamer, C.; de Beco, V.; Soler, P.; Calvat, S.; Fagon, J. Y.; Dombret, M. C.; Farinotti, R.; Chastre, J. and Gibert, C. "Analysis of vancomycin entry into pulmonary lining fluid by bronchoalveolar lavage in critically ill patients," *Antimicrob. Agents Chemother.*, vol. 37, no. 2, pp. 281–286, Feb. 1993.

[34] Moise, P. A.; Forrest, A.; Bhavnani, S. M.; Birmingham, M. C. and Schentag, J. J. "Area under the inhibitory curve and a pneumonia scoring system for predicting outcomes of vancomycin therapy for respiratory infections by Staphylococcus aureus," *Am. J. Heal.-Syst. Pharm. Ajhp Off. J. Am. Soc. Heal.-Syst. Pharm.*, vol. 57 Suppl 2, pp. S4–9, Oct. 2000.

[35] Malangoni, M. A.; Crafton, R. and Mocek, F. C. "Pneumonia in the surgical intensive care unit: factors determining successful outcome," *Am. J. Surg.*, vol. 167, no. 2, pp. 250–255, Feb. 1994.

[36] Wunderink, R. G.; Rello, J.; Cammarata, S. K.; Croos-Dabrera, R. V. and Kollef, M. H. "Linezolid vs vancomycin: analysis of two double-blind studies of patients with methicillin-resistant Staphylococcus aureus nosocomial pneumonia," *Chest*, vol. 124, no. 5, pp. 1789–1797, Nov. 2003.

[37] Rubinstein, E.; Cammarata, S.; Oliphant, T. and Wunderink, R. "Linezolid (PNU-100766) versus vancomycin in the treatment of hospitalized patients with nosocomial pneumonia: a randomized, double-blind, multicenter study," *Clin. Infect. Dis. Off. Publ. Infect. Dis. Soc. Am.*, vol. 32, no. 3, pp. 402–412, Feb. 2001.

[38] Wunderink, R. G.; Cammarata, S. K.; Oliphant, T. H. and Kollef, M. H. "Continuation of a randomized, double-blind, multicenter study of linezolid versus vancomycin in the treatment of patients with

nosocomial pneumonia," *Clin. Ther.*, vol. 25, no. 3, pp. 980–992, Mar. 2003.

[39] Walkey, A. J.; O'Donnell, M. R. and Wiener, R. S. "Linezolid vs glycopeptide antibiotics for the treatment of suspected methicillin-resistant Staphylococcus aureus nosocomial pneumonia: a meta-analysis of randomized controlled trials," *Chest*, vol. 139, no. 5, pp. 1148–1155, May 2011.

[40] Wunderink, R. G.; Niederman, M. S.; Kollef, M. H.; Shorr, A. F.; Kunkel, M. J.; Baruch, A.; McGee, W. T.; Reisman, A. and Chastre, J. "Linezolid in Methicillin-Resistant Staphylococcus aureus Nosocomial Pneumonia: A Randomized, Controlled Study," *Clin. Infect. Dis.*, vol. 54, no. 5, pp. 621–629, Jan. 2012.

[41] Alaniz, C. and Pogue, J. M. "Vancomycin versus linezolid in the treatment of methicillin-resistant Staphylococcus aureus nosocomial pneumonia: implications of the ZEPHyR trial," *Ann. Pharmacother.*, vol. 46, no. 10, pp. 1432–1435, Oct. 2012.

[42] Kullar, R.; Davis, S. L.; Levine, D. P. and Rybak, M. J. "Impact of Vancomycin Exposure on Outcomes in Patients With Methicillin-Resistant Staphylococcus aureus Bacteremia: Support for Consensus Guidelines Suggested Targets," *Clin. Infect. Dis.*, vol. 52, no. 8, pp. 975–981, Apr. 2011.

[43] Cataldo, M. A.; Tacconelli, E.; Grilli, E.; Pea, F.; and Petrosillo, N. "Continuous versus intermittent infusion of vancomycin for the treatment of Gram-positive infections: systematic review and meta-analysis," *J. Antimicrob. Chemother.*, vol. 67, no. 1, pp. 17–24, Oct. 2011.

[44] Wysocki, M.; Delatour, F.; Faurisson, F.; Rauss, A.; Pean, Y.; Misset, B.; Thomas, F.; Timsit, J. F.; Similowski, T.; Mentec, H.; Mier, L. and Dreyfuss, D. "Continuous versus intermittent infusion of vancomycin in severe Staphylococcal infections: prospective multicenter randomized study," *Antimicrob. Agents Chemother.*, vol. 45, no. 9, pp. 2460–2467, Sep. 2001.

[45] De Waele, J. J.; Danneels, I.; Depuydt, P.; Decruyenaere, J.; Bourgeois, M. and Hoste, E. "Factors associated with inadequate early vancomycin levels in critically ill patients treated with continuous infusion," *Int. J. Antimicrob. Agents*, vol. 41, no. 5, pp. 434–438, May 2013.

[46] Roberts, J. A.; Taccone, F. S.; Udy, A. A.; Vincent, J-L.; Jacobs, F.; Lipman, J. Vancomycin dosing in critically ill patients: robust methods

for improved continuous-infusion regimens. Antimicrob Agents Chemother. 2011;55(6):2704–2709. doi:10.1128/AAC.01708-10

[47]   Chastre, J.; Wolff, M.; Fagon, J.-Y.; Chevret, S.; Thomas, F.; Wermert, D.; Clementi, E.; Gonzalez, J.; Jusserand, D.; Asfar, P.; Perrin, D.; Fieux, F. and Aubas, S. "Comparison of 8 vs 15 days of antibiotic therapy for ventilator-associated pneumonia in adults: a randomized trial," *Jama J. Am. Med. Assoc.*, vol. 290, no. 19, pp. 2588–2598, Nov. 2003.

[48]   Bouadma, L.; Luyt, C.-E.; Tubach, F.; Cracco, C.; Alvarez, A.; Schwebel, C.; Schortgen, F.; Lasocki, S.; Veber, B.; Dehoux, M.; Bernard, M.; Pasquet, B.; Régnier, B.; Brun-Buisson, C.; Chastre, J. and Wolff, M. "Use of procalcitonin to reduce patients' exposure to antibiotics in intensive care units (PRORATA trial): a multicentre randomised controlled trial," *The Lancet*, vol. 375, no. 9713, pp. 463–474, Feb. 2010.

In: Vancomycin
Editor: Abu Gafar Hossion

ISBN: 978-1-62948-559-1
© 2013 Nova Science Publishers, Inc.

Chapter 8

Clinical Use of Vancomycin in Methicillin-Resistant Staphylococci Bone and Joint Infection

Florent Valour[1,2,3], Anissa Bouaziz[1,3],
Judith Karsenty[1,2], Thomas Barba[1],
Sandrine Leroy[1], Alicia Marquet[1],
Julien Saison[1,2], Frédéric Laurent[2,3,4],
Sébastien Lustig[3,5], Christian Chidiac[1,2,3]
and Tristan Ferry[1,2,3],*

[1]Infectious diseases department, Croix-Rousse Hospital,
Hospices Civils de Lyon, France
[2]Centre International de Recherche en Infectiologie, CIRI, Inserm U1111,
CNRS UMR5308, ENS de Lyon, UCBL1, Lyon, France
[3]Université Claude Bernard Lyon 1, Lyon, France
[4]Bacteriology Laboratory, Croix-Rousse Hospital,
Hospices Civils de Lyon, France
[5]Department of orthopaedic surgery, Centre Albert Trillat,
Croix-Rousse Hospital, Hospices Civils de Lyon, France

---

* Corresponding author: Tristan Ferry – Infectious Diseases department, Croix-rousse Hospital, 103 Grande-Rue de la Croix-Rousse, 69004 Lyon, France. Email: tristan.ferry@univ-lyon1.fr.

Abstract

In this chapter the clinical use of vancomycin in methicillin-resistant *S. aureus* or coagulase-negative staphylococci bone and joint infection (BJI) has been developed. BJI is one of the most difficult-to-treat infectious diseases, especially if an implant, such as osteosynthesis or joint prosthesis, is localized at the site of infection. These pathogens are the most frequent causative agents of BJI, particularly in postoperative or posttraumatic BJI. Staphylococci have the ability to modify their phenotype, by producing biofilm or small colony variants, which are particularly associated with chronic infection and relapse. In postoperative or in posttraumatic BJI, vancomycin has not to be used before optimal surgery (lavage and debridement, with implant retention or explantation), that: (i) allows the microbiological diagnosis; (ii) reduces the bacterial inoculum; (iii) eradicates sequestra in which staphylococci are embedded in biofilm; and (iv) facilitates bone vascularization and the diffusion of antimicrobials. Vancomycin has to be administered intravenously, through a central venous catheter (a peripheral access could be used during the first days of therapy), with a dosage of 15 mg/kg/d twice a day. As vancomycin activity is considered to be time-dependent, some data support the use of continuous infusion of vancomycin, to achieve a time under MIC (t/MIC) close to 100%. Targeting methicillin-resistant *S. aureus* or coagulase-negative staphylococci, vancomycin has to be combined with another active drug, and especially an oral drug, which has a high biodisponibility and bone penetration such as fluoroquinolones, clindamycin or rifampin. Rifampin has to be preferred in patients with implant-associated BJI. If possible, vancomycin could be switched after 2 weeks of therapy, to use a combination of two oral active drugs. If not, the regiment including vancomycin has to be prolonged until 6-24 weeks, depending on the clinical presentation. In these patients, it is crucial to monitor vancomycin trough serum concentration and to be aware of putative vancomycin toxicity.

Keywords: Vancomycin, bone and joint, infection

Introduction

BJI is one of the most difficult-to-treat infectious diseases, especially if an implant, such as osteosynthesis or prosthesis, is localized at the site of infection [1]. Staphylococci (i.e. *S. aureus* and coagulase-negative staphylococci) are the most frequent causative agents of BJI, with a prevalence reaching four quarter of cases in postoperative or posttraumatic BJI [1]. As other environmental bacteria, staphylococci have the ability to modify their phenotype to persist in hostile environment. In close contact with orthopaedic implants, it has been demonstrated that staphylococci has the ability to adhere and then to produce biofilm, which is a conglomeration of bacteria embedded within a self-produced extracellular matrix [2]. Staphylococci can also produce biofilm in sequestra, which is a dead ischemic bone that could be observed in patients with chronic osteomyelitis [1]. Once formed, the biofilm is inseparable from material, and the only possible way to heal is to explant the material, and to receive adapted antimicrobial therapy [1, 2, 3, 4]. Recently, it has been demonstrated that staphylococci exhibit a second way for persisting *in vivo*. Indeed, staphylococci and especially *S. aureus* invade and persist intracellularly within non-phagocytic cells, and especially synoviocytes and osteoblasts [5, 6]. Life in biofilm and intracellular persistence could be associated with the emergence of "small colony variants" that are detectable on blood agar culture media. These mechanisms associated with bacterial persistence probably explained why chronicity and relapse are frequently observed in patients with staphylococci BJI [3, 5, 6]. In a patient with BJI, teamwork is required to determine the best medicosurgical strategy, especially if the patient has a postoperative BJI such as implant-associated BJI [1, 3, 7]. During implant-associated infection, a surgical therapy is always required to: (i) allow the microbiological diagnosis; (ii) reduce the bacterial inoculum; (iii) eradicate sequestra in which staphylococci are embedded in biofilm; and (iv) facilitates the bone vascularization and the penetration of antimicrobials [1, 3, 7]. In patients with acute implant-associated infection (i.e. less than 1 month after the onset of symptoms), the implant could be retained but in patients with chronic infection (i.e. more than 1 month after the onset of symptoms), explantation of the implant is generally required to eradicate biofilm, and to limit the risk of relapse [1, 3, 7].

In postoperative or in posttraumatic BJI, vancomycin (as other antimicrobials) has not to be used before optimal surgery, as it may inhibit the bacterial growth in culture media, and hinder the bacterial diagnosis. Conversely, regarding to the high prevalence of staphylococci among BJI causative agents, the inclusion of antistaphylococcal in empirical therapy is of crucial importance following the bone sampling for microbiological cultures. Vancomycin remained the drug of choice in this indication, as it is efficient to inhibit both methicillin-susceptible and methicillin-resistant staphylococci [1,

3, 7]. Vancomycin has to be started in the operating room, intravenously, through a central venous catheter (a peripheral access could be used during the first days of therapy) with a perfusion of over 1 hour of 15 mg/kg/d twice a day. A beta-lactam such as ceftriaxone or piperacillin-tazobactam is usually associated with vancomycin as empirical therapy to target *Enterobacteriaceae*, which could be also involved in the process of infection, especially in patients with acute implant-associated infection [1, 3, 7].

Intermittent or Continuous Infusion of Vancomycin

There is a debate concerning vancomycin infusion modality during staphylococcal BJI. As vancomycin activity is mainly considered to be time-dependent, some data support the use of continuous infusion of vancomycin, to achieve a time under MIC (t/MIC) close to 100%. Recently, Dubée et al. published data about the use of continuous high-dose vancomycin therapy for methicillin-resistant staphylococcal prosthetic hip infection [8]. In this study, 60 patients received high doses of vancomycin, 40-60 mg/kg/day. Precisely, 20-30 mg/kg of vancomycin was dissolved in 50mL of 5% dextrose and administered continuously over a 12-h period twice daily via an infusion pomp. The target serum concentration was 30-40 mg/L, instead of the consensual target of 20 mg/L. For authors, several factors encourage the use of such doses: (i) coagulase-negative staphylococci are frequently heteroresistant to glycopeptides (i.e. susceptible to vancomycin, but resistant to teicoplanin) with high vancomycin minimal inhibitory concentration (MIC) in the range of susceptibility around 2-4 mg/L [3, 9, 10]; (ii) the vancomycin MIC obtained in vitro is underestimate as it could be higher at the site of infection under anaerobic condition; and (iii) the penetration of vancomycin into uninfected cortical bone is low, about 20-30% [11]. Ninteen patients (18.3%), "only", experienced nephrotoxicity, which was generally mild and reversible. Authors concluded that continuous high-dose intravenous vancomycin combination therapy was an effective, feasible and reasonably safe for patients with chronic methicillin-resistant staphylococci prosthesis joint infection. Previous cohort studies already suggested that continuous vancomycin infusion in high-dose therapy would be practical, effective and potentially safe [12, 13]. Recently, probably by considering that there was a lack of data on the safety of a such therapy (Elyasi et. al. found that patients receiving >30mg/kg/day of vancomycin are at high risk of nephrotoxicity), the IDSA guidelines for the diagnosis and management of prosthetic joint infection maintained the usual use of vancomycin, as previously described, i.e. 30 mg/kg/day in 2 intermittent perfusions [7, 15]. Of note, Cataldo et al. found in a meta-analysis that continuous perfusion reduce the risk of nephrotoxicity, in comparion with intermittent perfusion [16].

Use of Vancomycin as Definite Therapy

Clinical and Therapy Drug Monitoring

During vancomycin therapy, it is required to perform clinical monitoring to detect therapy-associated complications such as rash, signs of catheter infection, and thombosis.

Therapy drug monitoring, at least weekly, is required to target vancomycin trough serum concentration of at least 20 mg/L. A higher vancomycin serum concentration (25 or 30 mg/L) could be required, if the vancomycin MIC of the staphylococci is high in the range of susceptibility (i.e. 2 mg/L for *S. aureus* and 4 mg/L for coagulase-negative staphylococci). Usual laboratory testing such as blood cell count and creatinine blood level is also required to detect adverse reaction and toxicity.

Combination Antimicrobial Therapy

Receiving the results of bacterial cultures after sampling in the first 2 weeks, the physician has to combine vancomycin with another active drug, depending on the susceptibility testing. Targeting methicillin-resistant *S. aureus* or coagulase-negative staphylococci, vancomycin has to be combined with another active drug, and especially an oral drug, which has a high biodisponibility and bone penetration such as fluoroquinolones, clindamycin or rifampin [7]. Indeed, in a retrospective study on patients with methicillin-resistant *S. aureus* implant-associated orthopaedic infection, the use of vancomycin as single-agent antimicrobial therapy (in comparison with different drug combinations) was independently associated with treatment failure [14].

In addition to vancomycin, rifampin is the companion drug of choice in patients with implant-associated BJI, as rifampin is also effective on bacteria embedded in biofilm [1, 3, 7]. Despite, some authors reports an antagonism between rifampin and vancomycin in vitro, numerous animal models support the use of such combination [10, 17]. The rifampin introduction has to be delayed until obtaining: (i) the complete susceptibility testing of the strain; and (ii) optimal vancomycin concentrations in plasma; as: (i) some methicillin-resistant coagulase-negative staphylococci are rifampin resistant; and (ii) acquisition of rifampin resistance occurs quickly if the combination therapy is not effective [1, 3, 7, 18]. Depending on the pathogen drug's susceptibility, vancomycin could be switched after 2 weeks of therapy, if it's possible to combine rifampin with another active drug that could be administered orally. If not, the combination therapy including vancomycin has to be prolonged until 6-24 weeks, depending on the clinical presentation [1, 2, 3, 4, 5, 6, 7]. Due to the growing incidence of multidrug resistance in methicillin-resistant staphylococci, combination of vancomycin with an oral antibiotic is sometimes not possible. As a consequence, vancomycin has to be combined with another active drug, and fosfomycin could be an option. Indeed, recently, some authors demonstrated that in vitro, the combination vancomycin-fosfomycin has an enhanced bactericidal effect, even on high-inoculum or biofilm embedded methicillin-resistant *S. aureus* with vancomycin MIC equal to 2mg/mL [19]. This combination was used in the following case report.

Case Report

We report here the case of a patient with multidrug-resistant coagulase-negative staphylococci prosthesis joint infection treated with the combination vancomycin-fosfomycin. A 80-year-old woman with past history of *Staphylococcus lugdunensis* right knee prosthesis infection in 2001 (prosthesis implantation in 1999) was admitted in our unit in 2011 with the diagnosis of chronic right knee prosthesis infection. The patient had suppurative fistula at the lower part of the scar (figure 1, panel A). X-ray revealed prosthesis loosening with tibial periprosthetic lucencies (figure 1, panel B). A two-stage exchange was scheduled, with insersion of a cimented spacer after prosthesis explantation figure 2, panel A). A multidrug-resistant *S. epidermidis* grew from synovial fluid and four bone samples. Based on initial drug susceptibility testing, the pathogen was only susceptible to vancomycin, fosfomycin, and linezolid, and subpopulation of this pathogen expressed the "small colony variant" phenotype on blood agar culture media (normal sized colonies of coagulase-negative staphylococci on figure 3, panel A; tiny slow-growing colonies of the same pathogen, expressing the small colony variant phenotype on figure 3, panel B). Teicoplanin was inactive, suggesting a glycopeptide heteroresistance phenotype. The patient received continuous intravenous infusion of vancomycin (2500 mg per day, i.e 30 mg/kg/day) and intermittent intravenous infusion fosfomycin (12 g per day in 3 injections). Vancomycin MIC susceptibility testing revealed a high MIC of 3 mg/L (cutoff for vancomycin sensitivity of 4 mg/L). As the patient had a mild reduction of glomerular filtration (creatinine clearance of 50 mL/min), vancomycin daily dose was reduced to 1200 mg/day to obtain plasma concentrations between 20 and 25 mg/L. As the patient had a large bone defect, cimented constrained prosthesis (figure 2, panel B) was used for prosthesis reimplantation, which was performed 6 weeks after explantation, and under vancomycin and fosfomycin therapy. Antimicrobial treatment was prolonged 4 months, totaling 6 weeks of intravenous antimicrobial therapy. During the follow-up, the outcome was favorable.

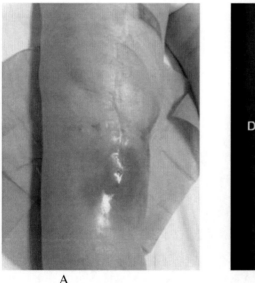 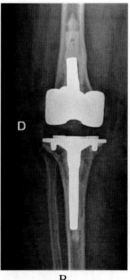

A   B

Figure 1. Case Report: Multidrug-resistant coagulase-negative staphylococci prosthesis joint infection treated with the combination vancomycin-fosfomycin towards 80-year-old woman (right knee prosthesis infection) with fistula (panel A), and prosthesis loosening (panel B).

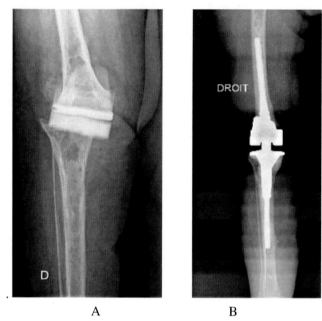

A   B

Figure 2. Case report: Multidrug-resistant coagulase-negative staphylococci prosthesis joint infection requiring prolonged antimicrobial therapy and a two-stage surgical procedure i.e. prosthesis explantation; a cement spacer was inserted to limit knee retraction (panel A), followed by a new prosthesis implantation several weeks later (panel B).

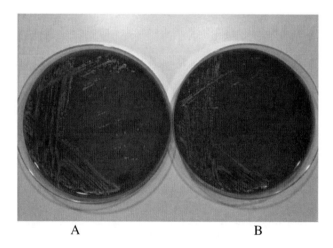

A   B

Figure 3. Pictorial view of normal sized colonies (panel A) and small colony variants (panel B) of the same coagulase-negative staphylococci.

Outpatient Parenteral Continuous Vancomycin Therapy

As patients with methicillin-resistant staphylococci BJI frequently required lengthy intravenous vancomycin infusion, they are eligible for outpatient parenteral antimicrobial therapy (OPAT) [20, 21]. Lengthy infusion of vancomycin at home required a central venous catheter, a teamwork approach (infectious disease physician with referring physician and nurse expert in intravenous therapy) and particular outcomes monitoring (treatment response, laboratory testing and prevention of therapy complications). Some authors previously described a high incidence of antimicrobial-related or catheter-related adverse event in patients receiving prolonged intravenous infusion of antibiotics [22, 23].

The large use since few years of peripheral inserted central catheter (PICC-line) reduce the risk of catheter-related complications, and especially immediate complication following the catheter infection. Vancomycin is easy to use during OPAT.

It could be infused twice daily, or continuously using a portable elastomeric infusion system (figure 4). OPAT offers several advantages: (i) reduction of the length of hospital stays; (ii) reduction of the cost in comparison with inpatient therapy; and (iii) the patient outcomes appear to be very good [20, 21].

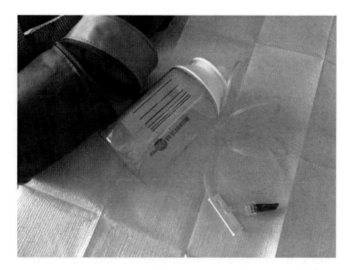

Figure 4. Elatomeric infusion system used for outpatient parenteral continuous vancomycin therapy.

Conclusion

Vancomycin is largely used in patients with methicillin-resistant staphylococci, as empirical therapy, but also frequently as definite therapy, in combination with rifampin or other active antistaphylococcal drug. Such patients are eligible for OPAT, with intermittent or continuous vancomycin infusion with elatomeric infusion system. Clinical and therapy drug monitoring is required during lengthy vancomycin therapy to detect vancomycin-associated complications.

Acknowledgments

This article was written on the behalf of the Lyon Bone and Joint Infection Study Group: *Lyon Bone and Joint Infection Study Group: Physicians* – Tristan Ferry, Thomas Perpoint, André Boibieux, François Biron, Florence Ader, Anissa Bouaziz, Judith Karsenty, Fatiha Daoud, Johanna Lippman, Evelyne Braun, Marie-Paule Vallat, Patrick Miailhes, Florent Valour, Christian Chidiac, Dominique Peyramond; *Surgeons* – Sébastien Lustig, Franck Trouillet, Philippe Neyret, Olivier Guyen, Gualter Vaz, Christophe Lienhart, Michel-Henry Fessy, Cédric Barrey, Pierre Breton; *Microbiologists* – Frederic Laurent, François Vandenesch, Jean-Philippe Rasigade; *Nuclear Medicine* – Isabelle Morelec, Marc Janier, Francesco Giammarile; *PK/PD specialists* – Michel Tod, Marie-Claude Gagnieu, Sylvain Goutelle; *Clinical Research Assistant* – Eugénie Marbut.

References

[1]   Lew, D. P.; Waldvogel, F. A. Osteomyelitis. *Lancet.* 2004 Jul 24-30; 364(9431): 369-79.
[2]   Montanaro, L.; Speziale, P.; Campoccia, D.; Ravaioli, S.; Cangini, I.; Pietrocola, G.; Giannini, S.; Arciola, C. R. Scenery of Staphylococcus implant infections in orthopedics. *Future Microbiol.* 2011 Nov; 6(11): 1329-49.
[3]   Trampuz, A.; Zimmerli, W. Diagnosis and treatment of implant-associated septic arthritis and osteomyelitis. *Curr. Infect. Dis. Rep.* 2008 Sep; 10(5): 394-403.

[4]   Evans, R. P.; Nelson, C. L.; Bowen, W. R.; Kleve, M. G.; Hickmon, S. G. Visualization of bacterial glycocalyx with a scanning electron microscope. *Clin. Orthop. Relat. Res.* 1998 Feb; (347): 243-9.

[5]   Sendi, P.; Rohrbach, M.; Graber, P.; Frei, R.; Ochsner, P. E.; Zimmerli, W. Staphylococcus aureus small colony variants in prosthetic joint infection. *Clin. Infect. Dis.* 2006 Oct 15; 43(8): 961-7. Epub 2006.

[6]   Valour, F. S.; Trouillet-Assant, J. P.; Rasigade, S.; Lustig, E.; Chanard, H.; Meugnier, S.; Tigaud, F.; Vandenesch, J.; Etienne, T.; Ferry, F. Laurent, on behalf of the Lyon BJI study group. *Staphylococcus epidermidis* in orthopedic device 1 infections: the role of bacterial internalization in human osteoblasts and biofilm formation. *PLoS One. 2013 In press.*

[7]   Osmon, D. R.; Berbari, E. F.; Berendt, A. R.; Lew, D.; Zimmerli, W.; Steckelberg, J. M.; Rao, N.; Hanssen, A.; Wilson, W. R. Diagnosis and management of prosthetic joint infection: clinical practice guidelines by the infectious diseases society of america. *Clin. Infect. Dis.* 2013 Jan; 56(1): e1-e25.

[8]   Dubée, V.; Zeller, V.; Lhotellier, L.; Kitzis, M. D.; Ziza, J. M.; Mamoudy, P.; Desplaces, N. Continuous high-dose vancomycin combination therapy for methicillin-resistant staphylococcal prosthetic hip infection: a prospective cohort study. *Clin. Microbiol. Infect.* 2013 Feb; 19(2): E98-105.

[9]   Vaudaux, P.; Ferry, T.; Uçkay, I.; François, P.; Schrenzel, J.; Harbarth, S.; Renzoni, A. Prevalence of isolates with reduced glycopeptide susceptibility in orthopedic device-related infections due to methicillin-resistant Staphylococcus aureus. *Eur. J. Clin. Microbiol. Infect. Dis.* 2012 Dec; 31(12): 3367-74.

[10] Saleh-Mghir, A.; Dumitrescu, O.; Dinh, A.; Boutrad, Y.; Massias, L.; Martin, E.; Vandenesch, F.; Etienne, J,; Lina, G.; Crémieux, A. C. Ceftobiprole efficacy in vitro against Panton-Valentine leukocidin production and in vivo against community-associated methicillin-resistant Staphylococcus aureus osteomyelitis in rabbits. *Antimicrob. Agents Chemother.* 2012 Dec; 56(12): 6291-7.

[11] Landersdorfer, C. B.; Bulitta, J. B.; Kinzig, M.; Holzgrabe, U.; Sörgel, F. Penetration of antibacterials into bone: pharmacokinetic, pharmacodynamic and bioanalytical considerations. *Clin. Pharmacokinet.* 2009; 48(2): 89-124.

[12] Boffi, E. l.; Amari, E.; Vuagnat, A.; Stern, R.; Assal, M.; Denormandie, P.; Hoffmeyer, P.; Bernard, L. High versus standard dose vancomycin for osteomyelitis. *Scand. J. Infect. Dis.* 2004; 36(10): 712-7.

[13] Vuagnat, A.; Stern, R.; Lotthe, A.; Schuhmacher, H.; Duong, M.; Hoffmeyer, P.; Bernard, L. High dose vancomycin for osteomyelitis: continuous vs. intermittent infusion. *J. Clin. Pharm. Ther.* 2004 Aug; 29(4): 351-7.

[14] Ferry, T.; Uçkay, I.; Vaudaux, P.; François, P.; Schrenzel, J.; Harbarth, S.; Laurent, F.; Bernard, L.; Vandenesch, F.; Etienne, J.; Hoffmeyer, P.; Lew, D. Risk factors for treatment failure in orthopedic device-related methicillin-resistant Staphylococcus aureus infection. *Eur. J. Clin. Microbiol. Infect. Dis.* 2010 Feb; 29(2):171-80.

[15] Elyasi, S.; Khalili, H.; Dashti-Khavidaki, S.; Mohammadpour, A. Vancomycin-induced nephrotoxicity: mechanism, incidence, risk factors and special populations. A literature review. *Eur. J. Clin. Pharmacol.* 2012; 68:1243-55.

[16] Cataldo, M. A.; Tacconelli, E.; Grilli, E.; Pea, F.; Petrosillo, N. Continuous versus intermittent infusion of vancomycin for the treatment of Gram-positive infections: systematic review and meta-analysis. *J. Antimicrob. Chemother.* 2012;67:17-24.

[17] Forrest, G. N.; Tamura, K. Rifampin combination therapy for nonmycobacterial infections. *Clin. Microbiol. Rev.* 2010 Jan; 23(1): 14-34.

[18] Achermann, Y.; Eigenmann, K.; Ledergerber, B.; Derksen, L.; Rafeiner, P.; Clauss, M.; Nüesch, R.; Zellweger, C.; Vogt, M.; Zimmerli, W. Factors associated with rifampin resistance in staphylococcal periprosthetic joint infections (PJI): a matched case-control study. *Infection.* 2013 Apr; 41(2): 431-7.

[19] Tang, H. J.; Chen, C. C.; Ko, W. C.; Yu, W. L.; Chiang, S. R.; Chuang, Y. C. In vitro efficacy of antimicrobial agents against high-inoculum or biofilm-embedded meticillin-resistant Staphylococcus aureus with vancomycin minimal inhibitory concentrations equal to 2 μg/mL (VA2-MRSA). *Int. J. Antimicrob. Agents.* 2011 Jul; 38(1):46-51.

[20] Tice, A. D.; Rehm, S. J.; Dalovisio, J. R.; Bradley, J. S.; Martinelli, L. P.; Graham, D. R.; Gainer, R. B.; Kunkel, M. J.; Yancey, R. W.; Williams, D. N; IDSA. Practice guidelines for outpatient parenteral antimicrobial therapy. IDSA guidelines. *Clin. Infect. Dis.* 2004 Jun 15; 38(12): 1651-72.

[21] Chapman, A. L.; Seaton, R. A.; Cooper, M. A.; Hedderwick, S.; Goodall, V.; Reed, C.; Sanderson, F.; Nathwani, D; BSAC/BIA OPAT Project Good Practice Recommendations Working Group. Good practice recommendations for outpatient parenteral antimicrobial therapy (OPAT) in adults in the UK: a consensus statement. *J. Antimicrob. Chemother.* 2012 May; 67(5): 1053-62.

[22] Pulcini, C.; Couadau, T.; Bernard, E.; Lorthat-Jacob, A.; Bauer, T.; Cua, E.; Mondain, V.; Chichmanian, R. M.; Dellamonica, P.; Roger, P. M. Adverse effects of parenteral antimicrobial therapy for chronic bone infections. *Eur. J. Clin. Microbiol. Infect. Dis.* 2008 Dec; 27(12): 1227-32.

[23] Duggal, A.; Barsoum, W.; Schmitt, S. K. Patients with prosthetic joint infection on IV antibiotics are at high risk for readmission. *Clin. Orthop. Relat. Res.* 2009 Jul; 467(7): 1727-31.

Index

Q

R